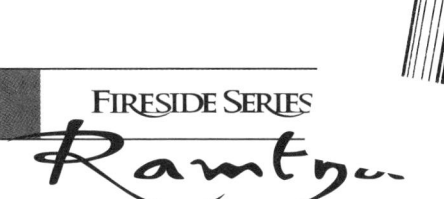

FIRESIDE SERIES

Ramtha

From Sexual Revolution
To God Revolution

FROM SEXUAL REVOLUTION
TO GOD REVOLUTION

Copyright © 2001 JZK, Inc.

Cover illustration by Carmel Bartz

All rights reserved. Printed in the United States of America. No part of this publication may be reproduced or transmitted in any form or by any means, electronic or mechanical, including photocopying, recording, or by any information storage and retrieval system, without the written permission of JZK Publishing, a division of JZK, Inc.

The contents of this publication are based on Ramtha Dialogues®, a series of magnetic tape recordings registered with the United States Copyright Office, with permission from JZ Knight and JZK, Inc. Ramtha Dialogues® and Ramtha® are trademarks registered with the United States Patent and Trademark Office.

This work is based on the partial transcription of Ramtha Dialogues®, Tape 374, *A Teaching Dedicated to the Feminine Gender and Understanding Molecules of Intent and Becoming a Christ*, February 3-7, 1998. Copyright ℗1998 JZK, Inc.

ISBN # 1-57873-060-0

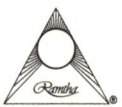

JZK Publishing,
A Division of JZK, Inc.

P.O. Box 1210
Yelm, Washington 98597
360.458.5201
800.347.0439
www.ramtha.com
www.jzkpublishing.com

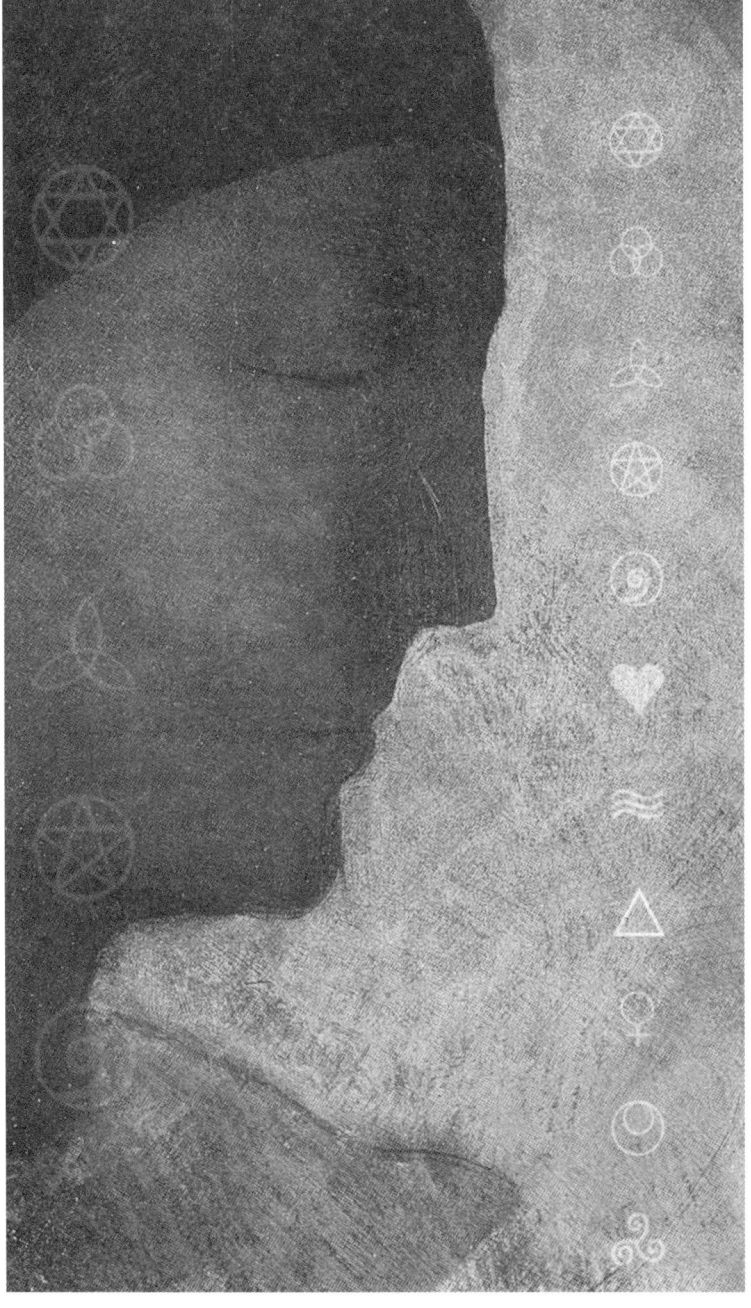

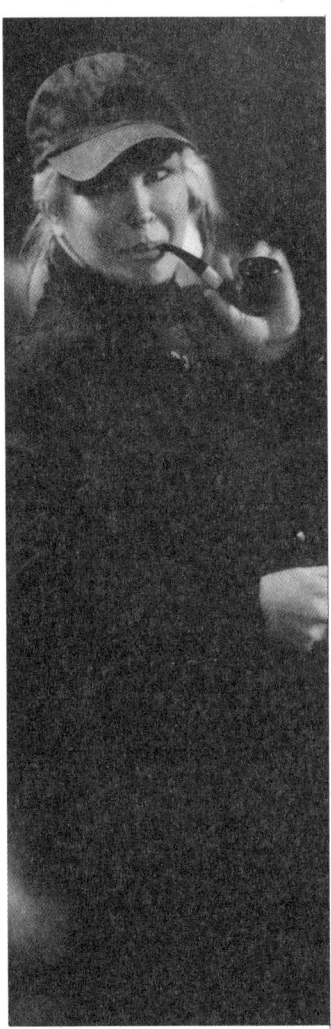

These series of teachings are designed for all the students of the Great Work who love the teachings of the Ram.

It is suggested that you create an ideal learning environment for study and contemplation.

Light your fireplace and get cozy. Have your wine and fine tobacco. Prepare yourself. Open your mind to learn and be genius.

FOREWORD TO THE NEW EDITION

The Fireside Series Collection Library is an ongoing library of the hottest topics of interest taught by Ramtha. These series of teachings are designed for all the students of the Great Work who love the teachings of the Ram. This library collection is also intended as a continuing learning tool for the students of Ramtha's School of Enlightenment and for everyone interested and familiar with Ramtha's teachings. In the last twenty-five years, Ramtha has continuously and methodically deepened and expanded his exposition of the nature of reality and its practical application through various disciplines. It is assumed by the publisher that the reader has attended a Beginning Retreat or workshop through Ramtha's School of Enlightenment or is at least familiar with Ramtha's instruction to his beginning class of students. This required information for beginning students is found in *Ramtha, A Beginner's Guide to Creating Reality*, revised and expanded ed. (Yelm: JZK Publishing, a division of JZK, Inc., 2000), and in *Ramtha: Creating Personal Reality*, Video ed. (Yelm: JZK Publishing, a division of JZK, Inc., 1998).

We have included in the Fireside Series a glossary of some of the basic concepts used by Ramtha so the reader can become familiarized with these teachings. We have also included a brief introduction of Ramtha by JZ Knight that describes how all this began. Enjoy your learning and contemplation.

CONTENTS

Introduction to Ramtha
By JZ Knight

"In other words, his whole point of focus is to come here and to teach you to be extraordinary."

You don't have to stand for me. My name is JZ Knight and I am the rightful owner of this body, and welcome to Ramtha's school, and sit down. Thank you.

So we will start out by saying that Ramtha and I are two different people, beings. We have a common reality point and that is usually my body. I am a lot different than he is. Though we sort of look the same, we really don't look the same.

What do I say? Let's see. All of my life, ever since I was a little person, I have heard voices in my head and I have seen wonderful things that to me in my life were normal. And I was fortunate enough to have a family or a mother who was a very psychic human being, who sort of never condemned what it was that I was seeing. And I had wonderful experiences all my life, but the most important experience was that I had this deep and profound love for God, and there was a part of me that understood what that was. Later in my life I went to church and I tried to understand God from the viewpoint of religious doctrine and had a lot of difficulty with that because it was sort of in conflict with what I felt and what I knew.

Ramtha has been a part of my life ever since I was born, but I didn't know who he was and I didn't know what he was, only that there was a wonderful force that walked with me, and when I was in trouble — and had a lot of pain in my life growing up — that I always had extraordinary experiences with this being who would talk to me. And I could hear him as clearly as I can hear you if we were to have a conversation. And he helped me to understand a lot of things in my life that were sort of beyond the normal scope of what someone would give someone as advice.

It wasn't until 1977 that he appeared to me in my kitchen on a Sunday afternoon as I was making pyramids with my husband at that time, because we were into dehydrating food and we were into hiking and backpacking and all that stuff. And so I put one of these ridiculous things on my head, and at the other end of my kitchen this wonderful apparition appeared that was seven feet tall and glittery and beautiful and stark. You just don't expect at 2:30 in the afternoon that this is going to appear in your kitchen. No one is ever prepared for that. And so Ramtha at that time really made his appearance known to me.

The first thing I said to him — and I don't know where this comes from — was that "You are so beautiful. Who are you?"

And he has a smile like the sun. He is extraordinarily handsome. And he said, "My name is Ramtha the Enlightened One, and I have come to help you over the ditch." Being the simple person that I am, my immediate reaction was to look at the floor because I thought maybe something had happened to the floor, or the bomb was being dropped; I didn't know.

And it was that day forward that he became a constant in my life. And during the year of 1977 a lot of interesting things happened, to say the least. My two younger children at that time got to meet Ramtha and got to experience some incredible phenomena, as well as my husband.

Later that year, after teaching me and having some difficulty telling me what he was and me understanding, one day he said to me, "I am going to send you a runner that will bring you a set of books, and you read them because then you will know what I am." And those books were called the *Life and Teachings of the Masters of the Far East* (DeVorss & Co. Publishers, 1964). And so I read them and I began to understand that Ramtha was one of those beings, in a way. And that sort of took me out of the are-you-the-devil-or-are-you-God sort of category that was plaguing me at the time.

And after I got to understand him, he spent long, long moments walking into my living room, all seven feet of this beautiful being making himself comfortable on my couch, sitting down and talking to me and teaching me. And what

I didn't realize at that particular time was he already knew all the things I was going to ask and he already knew how to answer them. But I didn't know that he knew that.

So he patiently since 1977 has dealt with me in a manner by allowing me to question not his authenticity but things about myself as God, teaching me, catching me when I would get caught up in dogma or get caught up in limitation, catching me just in time and teaching me and walking me through that. And I always said, "You know, you are so patient. You know, I think it is wonderful that you are so patient." And he would just smile and say that he is 35,000 years old, what else can you do in that period of time? So it wasn't really until about ten years ago that I realized that he already knew what I was going to ask and that is why he was so patient. But as the grand teacher that he is, he allowed me the opportunity to address these issues in myself and then gave me the grace to speak to me in a way that was not presumptuous but in a way, as a true teacher would, that would allow me to come to realizations on my own.

Channeling Ramtha since late 1979 has been an experience, because how do you dress your body for — Ram is seven feet tall and he wears two robes that I have always seen him in. Even though they are the same robe, they are really beautiful so you never get tired of seeing them. The inner robe is snow white and goes all the way down to where I presume his feet are, and then he has an overrobe that is beautiful purple. But you should understand that I have really looked at the material on these robes and it is not really material. It is sort of like light. And though the light has a transparency to them, there is an understanding that what he is wearing has a reality to it.

Ramtha's face is cinnamon-colored skin, and that is the best way I can describe it. It is not really brown and it is not really white and it is not really red; it is sort of a blending of that. And he has very deep black eyes that can look into you and you know you are being looked into. He has eyebrows that look like wings of a bird that come high on his brow. He has a very square jaw and a beautiful mouth, and when he smiles you know that you are in heaven. He has long, long hands, long fingers that he uses very eloquently to demonstrate his thought.

Well, imagine then how after he taught me to get out of my body by actually pulling me out and throwing me in the tunnel, and hitting the wall of light, bouncing back, and realizing my kids were home from school and I just got through doing breakfast dishes, that getting used to missing time on this plane was really difficult, and I didn't understand what I was doing and where I was going. So we had a lot of practice sessions.

You can imagine if he walked up to you and yanked you right out of your body and threw you up to the ceiling and said now what does that view look like, and then throwing you in a tunnel — and perhaps the best way to describe it is it is a black hole into the next level — and being flung through this tunnel and hitting this white wall and having amnesia. And you have to understand, I mean, he did this to me at ten o'clock in the morning and when I came back off of the white wall it was 4:30. So I had a real problem in trying to adjust with the time that was missing here. So we had a long time in teaching me how to do that, and it was fun and frolic and absolutely terrifying at moments.

But what he was getting me ready to do was to teach me something that I had already agreed to prior to this incarnation, and that my destiny in this life was not just to marry and to have children and to do well in life but to overcome the adversity to let what was previously planned happen, and that happening including an extraordinary consciousness, which he is.

Trying to dress my body for Ramtha was a joke. I didn't know what to do. The first time we had a channeling session I wore heels and a skirt and, you know, I thought I was going to church. So you can imagine, if you have got a little time to study him, how he would appear dressed up in a business suit with heels on, which he has never

14

walked in in his life.

But I guess the point that I want to tell you is that it is really difficult to talk to people — and perhaps someday I will get to do that with you, and understanding that you have gotten to meet Ramtha and know his mind and know his love and know his power — and how to understand that I am not him, and though I am working diligently on it, that we are two separate beings and that when you talk to me in this body, you are talking to me and not him. And sometimes over the past decade or so, that has been a great challenge to me in the public media because people don't understand how it is possible that a human being can be endowed with a divine mind and yet be separate from it.

So I wanted you to know that although you see Ramtha out here in my body, it is my body, but he doesn't look anything like this. But his appearance in the body doesn't lessen the magnitude of who and what he is. And you should also know that when we do talk, when you start asking me about things that he said, I may not have a clue about what you are talking about because when I leave my body in a few minutes, I am gone to a whole other time and another place that I don't have cognizant memory of. And however long he spends with you today, to me that will maybe be about five minutes or three minutes, and when I come back to my body, this whole time of this whole day has passed and I wasn't a part of it. And I didn't hear what he said to you and I don't know what he did out here. When I come back, my body is exhausted and it is hard to get up the stairs sometimes to change to make myself more presentable for what the day is bringing me, or what is left of the day.

You should also understand as beginning students, one thing that became really obvious over the years, that he has showed me a lot of wonderful things that I suppose people who have never got to see them couldn't even dream of in their wildest dreams. And I have seen the twenty-third universe and I have met extraordinary beings and I have seen life come and go. I have watched generations be born and live and pass in a matter of moments. I have been exposed to historical events to help me to understand better what it was I needed to know. I have been allowed to walk beside my body in other lifetimes and watch how I was and who I was, and I have been allowed to see the other side of death. So these are cherished and privileged opportunities that somewhere in my life I earned the right to have them in my life. To speak of them to other people is, in a way, disenchanting because it is difficult to convey to people who have never been to those places what it is. And I try my best as a storyteller to tell them and still fall short of it.

But I know that the reason that he works with his students the way that he does is because also Ramtha never wants to overshadow any of you. In other words, his whole point of focus is to come here and to teach you to be extraordinary; he already is. And it is not about him producing phenomena. If he told you he was going to send you runners, you are going to get them big time. It is not about him doing tricks in front of you; that is not what he is. Those are tools of an avatar that is still a guru that needs to be worshiped, and that is not the case with him.

So what will happen is he will teach you and cultivate you and allow you to create the phenomenon, and you will be able to do that. And then one day when you are able to manifest on cue and you are able to leave your body and you are able to love, when it is to the human interest impossible to do that, one day he will walk right out here in your life because you are ready to share what he is. And what he is is simply what you are going to become. And until then he is diligent, patient, all-knowing, and all-understanding of everything that we need to know in order to learn to be that.

And the one thing I can say to you is that if you are interested in what you have heard in his presentation, and you are starting to love him even though you can't see him, that is a good sign because it means that what was important in you was your soul urging you to unfold in this lifetime. And it may be against your neuronet. Your personality can argue with you and debate with you, but you are going to learn that that sort of logic is really transparent when the soul urges you onto an experience.

And I can just say that if this is what you want to do, you are going to have to exercise patience and focus and you are going to have to do the work. And the work in the beginning is very hard. But if you have the tenacity to stay with it, then one day I can tell you that this teacher is going to turn you inside out. And one day you will be able to do all the remarkable things that in myth and legend that the masters that you have heard of have the capacity to do. You will be able to do them because that is the journey. And ultimately that ability is singularly the reality of a God awakening in human form.

Now that is my journey and it has been my journey all of my life. And if it wasn't important and if it wasn't what it was, I certainly wouldn't be living in oblivion most of the year for the sake of having a few people come and have a New Age experience. This is far greater than a New Age experience. And I should also say that it is far more important than the ability to meditate or the ability to do yoga. It is about changing consciousness all through our lives on every point and to be able to unhinge and unlimit our minds so that we can be all we can be.

You should also know that what I have learned is we can only demonstrate what we are capable of demonstrating. And if you would say, well, what is blocking me from doing that, the only block that we have is our lack to surrender, our ability to surrender, our ability to allow, and our ability to support ourself even in the face of our own neurological or neuronet doubt. If you can support yourself through doubt, then you will make the breakthrough because that is the only block that stands in your way. And one day you are going to do all these things and get to see all the things that I have seen and been allowed to see.

So I just wanted to come out here and show you that I exist and that I love what I do and that I hope that you are learning from this teacher and, more importantly, I hope you continue with it.

— *JZ Knight*

TRUE BEAUTY AND VALUE OF THE FEMININE GENDER

You made it. So be it. My beloved people, who are loved more than any people in this galaxy or any other, I salute you from the Lord God of my being to the Lord God of your being. I can't tell you in this language how happy I am to be back. I will tell you why — it should never be a why — but because those of you who were at the last Retreat have made great changes in your life and you are working on it. And don't you know that you are starting to send ripples on the pond of your life, and this makes me very happy? You are listening and you are doing.

This is what masters made up their mind to become the day they decided to no longer be the image of their past, and that was the key to mastership. When they were no longer what they thought themselves to be emotionally, the day they were free to create that which is termed new dreams and new paradigms without any emotion, waiting for the experience of that dream, then have the emotion, that is a master. And you are starting to learn.

I swear,
from the Lord God of my being,
that I shall love God
above all creatures,
all people,
places,
things,
times, and events.
And with this love
I shall be eternal.
I swear
that in God
I shall live forever,
and I will never forget.

I dedicate my life
to the adventure
of my Holy Spirit
and bury my past
on deserts dry
and never to revisit,
so help me God.
So be it.
To eternal life.

All women who are smoking pipes, you squeeze up here. Come on. I invited those who were smoking their pipe to join me because it is an unfeminine characteristic; it is reserved only for men. And yet the heaviest cigarette smokers are always women, because they are endeavoring not to find pleasure in that which is termed their tobacco but find equality. That is the only reason that they do it.

Now tonight's teaching not only is a coming together of love that loves love, which is you and I, but also a teaching before the entity who comes here tomorrow who is going to teach you in a scientific mode about the body. I want you to understand something: Science has not found all of the answers. And though you are going to understand that which is termed peptides as informational substance to that which is termed the body, I have taught you yet a greater, more righteous knowledge. If science was at this precipice, then there would be a whole mutation of the society in the West. That has not happened yet. It is happening in small pockets, in particularly this pocket.

Now so tonight I want to address that which is termed the feminine gender, and that is the reason why I have these pipe-smoking women in my presence. First off, I want you men to understand this. If I said tonight I was going to march on some place, and I had that in mind — But my daughter has cautiously told me from another plane not to say that word, so I am going to edit it. And you see this group that is sitting here on this stage? They would be warriors, amazons — yes, that is true — and they would march. They would march and, in with their tears, they would swing a sword.

Tonight is dedicated simply to that which is termed the female gender in understanding, in all these years that we have been together, that men and women are only that which is termed the mechanical vehicle for a God that is neither.

So now what did you see in the light before you came back here? You saw that which is termed a gender endeavoring to combine that which is termed compassion and love with strength. But strength has always been that which is termed the prerequisite to the man because the man was always that which went out and fought for the family's honor, which went out and fought the wild beasts of that which is termed the forest to bring home that which is termed foodstuffs. So the man actually always represented in every society the strength of the family union.

But if we take into consideration the strength that it takes of a woman from the fruit of the womb to usher forth in birth pains a new life, then we are talking about such pain that few men have ever, ever experienced. Now so when many entities say there are more women that are drawn to a new movement than men, there is truth in that because women have always possessed the side of strength, but unfortunately they have never been given that which is termed the permission to call it strength, because strength, as it were, to bring forth children into the world could never be measured in the masculine world. The masculine world only measures strength as to getting up every day and laboring into that which is termed the fields, to bring home the food to feed the family.

But the male never understood the female's worry, anxiousness, anxiety, and indomitable strength to bring forth children into the world. And they in one sense are closer to God because they know what it is to go inside and to expand themselves and to give of themselves that which is termed a new lifeform. Women were always considered the ultimate Goddess because they were the ones who ultimately on a matter-of-fact level turned inward and conceived and then brought outward that which is termed the fruit of the womb. How many of you understand? And so we understand that which is termed the understanding of nature, that nature is that which is termed a feminine gender because nature gives life and it takes away life. It is the woman who bears the responsibility of the new life. And of her body, her body is sapped of its vital life force to give that which is termed life to the new child that will come forth into a freed land.

So tonight we understand from the Observer's point of view the feminine. And from the feminine's point of view, as the Observer who gets to understand both parts of the polaric spectrum, we begin to see how the Observer set forth that which is termed not in the enjoyment of lust but the need of lust to reconcile that which is termed individual experience in a woman.

We see then that the power of the woman — fragile, much softer, much more "aqualine," much more beautiful than the features of a man — we saw that their bodies are soft. We saw that their bodies were able to that which is termed to produce and to carry a child, to receive the semen of a man, and to be able to enlarge itself to be able to support a child and then have that which is termed the downy softness of skin in which to cradle a new lifeform, as if we were being cradled in the bosom of God itself.

We see how the Observer then could choose in a life to be a woman, because in a woman we see softness, yet strength. We see beauty, yet sovereignty. We see that which is termed creativeness from the womb itself, that which is termed the Void re-creating itself.

So now why did man always fear woman? Because woman was never governed by the places that man in his first seal was, that woman was governed from a higher order naturally, and the higher order is survival. Whereas man, who cannot bear the heat of the forthcomingness of his seed, must have his way, a woman gives her way only because she sees that in the fortuitous sight of survival itself.

And a woman will give herself not in passion but in survival. A woman's ultimate root of passion is not passion but survival, whereas man, the ultimate root of passion is passion. How many of you understand? So be it.

So if women work from a greater point in the seals, then that means that their power place has always been the third seal, that they could control pain and sexuality as that which is termed recommended to them to their survival. Men could never control their first seal in survival. They never could. It was always the undoing of every man. It was his Achilles heel. A man who was weak in his first seal could always be conquered. I knew that in my lifetime. Don't you understand that we could send the greatest hetaera to that which is termed my greatest enemy and always find him weak, and the one enemy who wasn't weak to that was an enemy worthy of battle? Do you understand that? I knew that as a man.

Women, on the other hand, have a jump-start on evolution. Men are created to spill their seed every moment of the day that they are replenished. Women have only one cycle a month to which they are only that which is termed passion, and that passion is greatest when it is afforded their reproductive cycle. Any other time other than that, their passion is seduction, and their seduction is their power. How many of you understand?

I want you to pause for a moment and look at this. Look how many women I have around me. Even the most virile of you men and the most seductive of you men do not have this sort of audience. Well, my, my. I am only a personality in this woman's body. How do you account for this? What are they attracted to? Let me tell you a little secret, you old men of wise, sage belief: In my day all of these women would have gladly come to my tent. And even today I can love your women greater than you can. I can. I can. So what do I know that you do not know, my beloved fellow masters? What do I know you do not know? You look upon me and I am just a wee, little woman.

Now why? Because I considered them equal, I

considered that they were God. And the closer they acted like that, the more beautiful they were to me, and that anytime you look upon the God of a woman instead of her femininity — Her breasts, her vagina, her legs, her buttocks, her body, how much she weighs, how much she doesn't weigh, anytime that that becomes a standard of measurement to you, you have lost a very elevated entity. And they, of course, the elevated entity, doesn't know they are elevated because they have never been exposed to anything greater than what they can possibly get. Are you listening to me?

So how does a man make love to a woman? By loving her divinity above anything else — her face, her body, her breasts, her vagina, how she is in your bed — but to love that first and foremost because that speaks to the eternalness of her being because, after all, her isn't a her. Do you understand?

And most of you men in the audience, all you think about is how young a face is, how skinny the body is, how much breast there is, how much womb there is, how much, because you can only get one who is equal to your first seal. But it is yet now another challenge to have one who is equal to your third seal. And all women naturally are third-seal entities because in and of themselves they are not first-seal entities. They use the first seal as a place of power and only power. 'Tis a great truth.

So how indeed then must you start to change, my beloved men of this audience? And if any woman in this audience that is in the Great Work is worth her salt, she should never settle for one who will only placate her for the sake of her sexuality but will understand and communicate with her on the level of the divine and nothing but the divine, because when that is considered equal, everything else follows. To be less than that, if you ask a woman, "Love you this man," most of them will say yes. But if you have the vision to look at them, you will see that they tell you that because — they say that only because — it is for the children they have bore to this man, and that this man is not only the root of the survival of their children and/or the root of the survival of themselves, or they, as it were, will be the survivalist in the family so that the children can have their natural father.

Women, more than any other who are closest to the fourth seal, do not understand love because they have always had to anchor down to love to the first seal, the second seal, in order to make their way in life. And to have had a greater and a higher standard, their fears were always brought up about spinsterhood and ugliness and overweightedness and all of the silly things that you try to become for the sake of men. You have anchored down already your evolutionary step for that which is termed an image ideal that in the end is going to give way to the worm itself.

WHAT IS TRUE LOVE REALLY ABOUT?

Now the last Retreat you learned about that which is termed informational substances. You understood that that which is termed, as it were, the brain hath every peptide that can formulate in every receptor site in the body itself. So if the brain is self-contained, as it were, except for the mobility and the momentum to which the body offers to it — and to which the long torso that allows the digestive tract of nutrients to be broken down to feed the greatest crown of all, to serve this here[1] — then we have to look at this here and say what then lies as the paradigm of that which is termed true love.

Is true love about appearance? Is true love about that which is termed youth or age, or is true love that which is termed something that cannot be calibrated in the first three seals but is calibrated only in the fourth? And if we say that women use their passion to control and to seduce willing men who are willing only to be serviced — this is an ugly term, to service a man, and many of you do that — you service them so that you can keep yourself in their space of focus, all along denying the power of the place that you sit; that if you were able to love from that place of power, and you were able to garner to yourself first the recognition that you are God, and that maybe you have been a man and that you have been many times a woman, so who is it that we must then reconcile ourself to?

We were born into this plane as polaric entities, negative to positive, that attraction that is so strong that it is no wonder that the energy of that attraction sits in the first seal, that it sits in the first seal for the sake of propagation. But in ten and a half million years you have evolved somewhat to understand that though this can be

---

1 The brain.

recreational, it is not time-honored commitment, and that indeed the greatest mates of our being we will never be attracted to here[2] — we will be attracted to here[3] because it is God to God. This will always feel righteous but it will not feel the heat of this[4] in the beginning. If this is the heat in the beginning, then it is doomed because it can only replicate itself so far as to be bored with itself, because as long as there is a restless Spirit in men and women, they will never be happy with their partner. And why? Because their partner never really represents who they really are. And until you begin to seek out that which you really are, are you going to be filled in all the seals to which is the level of your own evolution.

What Does It Mean to Be a Woman?

Now tonight I want you to know that these women's emotional bodies are set and geared biologically and genetically, which we are talking about the DNA or gender here. They are geared for that which is termed survival, and children have always been a part of their survival, and if it has not been children, it has been the pleasure of sexuality. But most women have their greatest comfort sexually when they know that they have owned their man. I want you to understand it is a truth. And though they may gain pleasure from it, they work and labor specifically in which to become everything so sexually that they who labor so much, if you say to them, "Why do you work so hard on being beautiful; why do you work so hard on being thin; why do you work so hard on being a hetaera; why?" and the answer is "to keep my man happy," an enlightened being would look at that and say if you have to live your life for the momentary pleasure of a man, you are already dead. You are already dead. If you are having to live to

2 The first seal, sexual attraction.
3 The fourth seal, unconditional love.
4 The first seal.

capture a certain individual, that means you are dying to your enlightenment for the sake of the comfort of a person who is not equal to you. The day that women recognize that their equality is in God and not in men is the day they get to share the journey of men, who also see that their equality is in God and not in women, on the journey back home. So be it.

And if you have to gear down to someone and you have to deny to someone and you have to pretend to be something other than what you really are, that is not evolutionary. You are going to die, and you will be born again in this body with the same curse every twenty-one days until you realize what you are really here to be.

Now what does it mean to be a woman? It means that God is closer to being realized, because the womb of creation sits right below the fourth seal and that in realization we must make a decision: Are we going to then live our life as women, prone to our moods and indeed our bodies, are we going to live our life prone to the necessity of having someone make us feel great, or do we live our life first and foremost that we are God in a woman's body and delight in being the woman, delight in being beautiful, delight in being old, delight in having wisdom, delight in our bodies, and in that we are virtuous because then we are real? When we do that, then we are nearer to God. And we say then that this will eliminate 99.9 percent of the world's men from our life, then so be it. "I can walk this life alone and become nearer to my God." That is the way it is. Or to that which is termed a wonderful happiness, we find an opposite gender, a man, who has thought the same, who shares our life, and to eliminate them because of our prejudice is as much a backward manifestation as the one that we have struggled to come up from.

Now I have men and women here who are really Gods, the forgotten Gods. This body is a garment. Its emotions controlled you; that is why you came to school. You are here not to be better men and women but to finally be God, the most important thing. That is what a master is all about. A master has to be beautiful to no one but God. And it is not what we look like but how we are morally: our thoughts, our Observer. If our Observer can see the fallacy of our humanity, the day our Observer sees itself is the day we have arrived at godhood. In other words, the day that our Observer sees life without the positive or the negative is the day that our God has become ourself. That is the beginning of our Christhood.

Women cannot live their life for the sake of being a woman. And the day that their common thought becomes that of God instead of their feminine gender — in other words, the day that the Observer observes the Observer — is the day that we have immortal life. For women that is closer than for men. That is the reason why there are so many crossovers in the world, so many men in prior lives that have become women, because a woman is the path that is closest to redemption. 'Tis a truth.

And men have the longest, hardest journey of the two because their whole image is connected to their penis. Every part of their physical maturity is connected to their penis. Men have a hard time every day getting up and going through the day without ejaculation. Women don't have a problem. The day that the man no longer is connected to his penis but is connected to his fourth seal and works arduously to be that and can still consider himself a God, not a man, is the day that he is nearer to God and he is on the equal precipice with women.

Sexual Revolution and Freedom

Now there has certainly been in the twentieth century a revolution for women's liberation. And women's liberation gave them the permission to have multiple lovers and not feel guilty about it, and gave them the permission to have passion without the responsibility of children. And this then was dreamed into reality: for you to love many men and have no children, as you wished; to know what it was to be a man in previous lifetimes who had that ability to do that, a man who can love a woman and walk away from the fruit of her womb and from her. You have gotten in this century the opportunity to do that. That is not by accident; that was created. So with birth control came, as it were, your liberation to a greater point of degree to where you got to live your passionate life and explore it without responsibility. That is not a bad thing. That is an evolutionary evolvement.

Now most of you who got to see that have come to the shallow point that, as you were on an equal standard of men and women, got to understand that there is an emptiness and hollowness about that which is termed sexuality. And if you did, it is those of you who came to this school who said I have had the liberation to be all of these things but I am garnered to yet a higher degree of understanding. That higher degree of understanding says that I obviously chose this life and I obviously had the ability to choose this life to exercise my discretion in childbearing. Perhaps in this life I had the ability and I earned the ability to explore those forbidden areas, that — save for only hetaerae, who knew the science of cycles in women, did not have to have children — I can finally learn and explore those regions. Now that I have explored them, I have found that which is termed it is empty to lie with a man who loves me only for my body and is yet concerned not for my deeper thoughts, and yet it is my deeper thoughts that govern me and guide me throughout this life.

You got through your emotional body the freedom of sexual freedom without responsibility. When do you say then I know what that is; I know what it is to lie with a man without the responsibility of the man and indeed without the responsibility of his children? When do you have enough that you can say when is it then I can lie with God and have the responsibility of God? When then can I finally see this is so empty and here I am in the place that I have geared down forever and ever and ever from my place of power? Can I use power — which is will, manipulation, cleverness, stalwartness, frankness — can I use that same asset to catapult myself into a greater realm? And indeed am I willing to leave behind the world's men who are brought up in the nursery of the world, and can I leave it behind and perhaps on my way find a companion or find not a companion? That is what the master of women is all about.

Women need to understand that they are not less than men, and that they should never be property of men, and indeed that they should not feel that the only thing that is good about them is their uterus or their bosom or their buttocks, and that to think that is not to love yourself. I want you to know that. If you are endeavoring to live for the affections of a man by the way you look, then you are already dead and have never wakened up, because men traditionally live from their first seal.

But men's greatest competition is not women but it is men on the third seal in what is called competition. Men love to beat men at their own games — women are passive — in that which is termed only to have relief from the sperm that is built up in their loins. I want you to know that. And men take women so as to offer that which is termed an indignancy to their fellow man to say, "I got this woman and now you don't have them." It is the harem concept. Harem concept in mentality in men is old. It is old.

The day that my women say, "I am living for my God, and I will live from that morality, and indeed I will live from that beauty, and I will live from that clarity, and I will not sell my body short for any man who enters my sphere for the sake of making him feel grand, I will keep myself for my God," is a wise woman and a wise woman who will never sell herself short ever again to belong to a harem, because men are fickle. Men are fickle. When they live in their first seal, they can never be truthful. If they live in their fourth seal, they are honored by the stamp of God. It is this that you want and nothing else. You should no longer be less than what you have naturally always been.

And this speaks to all of the men in the audience, as well, who feel the same way. You should never feel that you need to leave that which is termed a higher order to play the game of a lower order. You don't need to do that. If you are not living your life for what society thinks about you, then it is time that you dispense with the fallacies of your life and start living a truism, start living righteously. Who cares what the world thinks? Who cares who you are with? Who cares if you are alone? Who cares what the men in your circle say? If you are on the path, that is all that matters to your God. Who cares what say they? And perhaps then that is your challenge and indeed that is your mastery.

I honor the women tonight because forever they have been herded like cattle into harems. They have been bought and sold. They have been taken into marriage only to be betrayed. The men who gave them their honor they would be true to them always lied, and it was understood that they could lie. But the women were never allowed to be anything other than their word.

I want my women in this audience who smoke pipes with me to understand they are liberated, and they are liberated not in a sexual liberation but in their God liberation, that they have lived ten and a half million years of life. Who haven't you been? What haven't you been in ten and a half million years? If you haven't been better than you think your dreams are, you have been uncreative in your past ten and a half million years.

Greatness, real greatness, that epic of memory: Who in this audience do you think is going to be remembered two thousand years from tonight? Do you think the most beautiful woman in this audience is going to be remembered two thousand years from now? They won't. Do you think the ugliest man in this audience is going to be remembered two thousand years from now? How about the most beautiful man in this audience; do you think he is going to be remembered two thousand years from now? Sorry, you don't register.

What is remembered? An entity who lives their truth, be it male or female — and females rarely. It is time that you become torches in the new millennium. It is true. I tell you your God in you is not prejudiced as gender is prejudiced. Your God chose you for a reason. You bring to the table of evolution opportunity, not sexuality. Remember that. Your God chose this body for opportunity and not sexuality. And if you do not create opportunity, master it, and are willing to own it as wisdom, then you will only go down in the graveyards of the West or the East as something that was remembered and smells badly. Do you understand? Will you turn to your partner and explain, kindly.

Is Sex a Wrong Thing?

So now we gathered together and we began to see how it is no wonder why there are more women who vacillate to the truth, because it is closer to them; it is what they really are. And whenever women can really apply the message, without going down and take it up, are the ones that go home very easily.

So, my beautiful women, is sexuality a wrong thing? No, it is not. But it becomes a disgrace to your honor as a God when you abuse it for the sake of survival; then it dishonors you. And you should never keep company with that which dishonors you — ever, ever. You are born nearer to God. From nearer to God you should go upward with it. And, yes, it is a very powerful test, especially when you are young or when you are about to lose that which is termed the blush of your maidenhood. Then you are panicked because what will the world think of you as that which is termed wrinkles and sags, and all of that starts in on your body; what will they think of you?

But you have to ask yourself who are you pursuing. Are you pursuing the youth of ignorance? Are you pursuing the wisdom of eternity? Young people don't know any better. Do you really want to give up your life for the sake of an inexperienced and ignorant person? A wise man or a wise woman would never do that. And do you want to panic that you are losing your youth? Now there is reason to panic because you have lived by your body's emotion for so long. What will happen when you look in the mirror and it is no longer beautiful when it looks back at you? What are you going to do?

But who are you being beautiful for, yourself or what the world thinks? If you live for what the world thinks, you are already dead. You will never hear anything else I have to say to you. But if you look at your beautiful self and cultivate all of the wisdom that you have learned, and if you can peel the onion, peel it until you find the core — why did I do this; I did it for this; why did I do that; I did it for that; and why did I do this; I did it for that — and if you can find the core of all of your reaction, you have found truth, and it will set you free.

How many times have you been women in the course of ten and a half million years? I would say more than fifty percent. How many times have you been young and beautiful? More than fifty percent. How many more times can you be that? More than fifty percent. When is the day that you take a chance and say, "Can I cultivate something other than physical wisdom — how about my mind? — and not settle for anything other than that which matches my mind?" The day that you do that is the day that you are awakened and nearer to God. The day you don't do that is when you are nearer to your femininity.

Women are awesome beings. Don't you know that the whole strategy of men for all of this time to enslave you and to mark you and to cattle you and to use you and abuse you is because you had a power because you were a law unto your own self? Don't you know that there was something to be afraid of there and to use? If you weren't anything that was threatening, you would never have been herded like cattle, never would have been, nor would have religion set out to permanently destroy who you are.

This business about Mary having children when she is a virgin, obviously a man of myth created that. You learn to be your own person and don't you ever trade your body for security. Don't you ever do that. Don't you ever do that.

You have done that many lifetimes. Don't you ever do that again. And don't you ever take someone to your bed that is less than you. Don't you ever do that. And you go about creating your enlightenment for the sake of you. Don't you know you are worthy to fall in love with? And don't you know that the long, dry spell of walking the path, that sooner or later some beautiful entity is going to join you who is also there?

Rare are masters. The reason that they are not rare is because of their sexuality. But that is why this is called the plane of demonstration. So is there that fear that as you have grown older you wasted your youth on a cattleman's idea or indeed that which is termed an idea that you threw away your youth and your volatility? You only have to have intercourse one time to understand what it is. After the hymen is broken, we should have wisdom.

Look, every event I watch you and I watch the games you play. You think that I miss anything? I don't miss anything. I know who is playing a game to get this person interested in them and that person interested in them. I know what you are doing. Don't you know? Of course you know. But did you ever stop and think that there was a knowingness that knew you were doing that? What about going after that knowingness? What can it offer you? Everything that you don't see in front of you. How many of you understand?

You are just fine without a man in your life. You are just fine. You really are. You are just as important and you are just as beautiful and you are natural. You are actually supernatural. You are just as important without your breasts and your vagina and your face because — think about this — the face and the breasts and the vagina become only a small part of life. Think about birth to death and what part of that are you really beautiful. How many years are you fertile and beautiful before you start to age? It is less than a third. What are you going to do with the rest of it? Are you going to live in regret and anger and unhappiness?

What you have to do is start now and say, "I am enough. I have always been enough," and you have to live for your ideal. You have to live for what gives you comfort and what gives you beauty and what gives you truth. You cannot rely on any man for truth. You have to rely on yourself. Furthermore, you cannot rely on any man to support you. You need to support yourself because to do anything otherwise is to have affairs and liaisons for the sake of survival and not for meaningful existence. How many of you understand? So be it.

THE FOCUS SHOULD BE
WHAT ARE YOU AS A MIND

Now, my beloved people, have you learned tonight? So what did this Retreat have to do with the last Retreat? Well, a lot. In the last Retreat we understood that that which is termed emotion and chemicals are the voices in your head. You also learned that that which talks to you up here has an ulterior motive, and the ulterior motive is emotion. It is only chemicals that talk to the neuronet. That is why it sounds like a voice. How many of you understand?

So most of you respond to the voices in your head because indeed you are responding to chemical emotion. Chemical emotion is a past; present has yet to be felt. We want to create a future-present; we create that which is termed a future that starts off with an ideal. The ideal, we should know, is not going to have any emotion, and the only thing we are going to feel, if feeling can be interpreted as the proper term, is the freedom to be able to create this concept. The concept is not going to feel like anything. You are addicted to feeling. New concepts don't feel any of these things. If anything, they feel like they are free. That is the path of the master.

Now listen to me, particularly my women. You are emotional beings because you have always gone backwards in order to refacilitate an emotion and consequently you have never grown in your life. You have always held to your bed that which was equal to a past, never what you really dreamed about being. When we create from the Observer, we should know whatever we create is not going to have an emotion with it. Women's tendency is to rush and find an emotion. I don't want you to do that. You know why I tell you it is your tendency to do that? Because your whole survival with men for a very long time genetically has been to find what makes them feel good. Men love it when you make them feel good, but they don't like it when you are not making

45

them feel good. And you have learned that.

So one of your great strategies is to create an emotional situation that the man can solve because that is who you go to with your emotional problems. But didn't you ever really listen, if you think about it, to the voice in your head that already knew the answer? You were playing a game, and you have always played games. The truth is you already knew the answer and you were putting on this play, and you have even watched yourself do it. You have watched yourself create unnecessary problems for solving by the other gender. That said it all. That has to be dispensed of, and it has to be dispensed of because you have got to stop being clever; you have got to start being real. You can always go down to the nearest welfare office to get food. You don't have to prostitute your intelligence for the sake of somebody giving you a meal, which you have always done. How many of you understand that? And you don't have to prostitute yourself to make the man feel better.

You may come to this wonderful realization that when you really become real — real — and just are who you are without playing any game, yes, you are going to have to maybe lose the person who is sharing your bed, but maybe the next person who shares your bed will be your equal. You understand?

And are there equals? Absolutely. Are there equals for men? Absolutely, because just as I am telling you this, there are men in this audience who already know the program. And they sell themselves out sexually because they understand the whole game. And they play the game because they are satisfied sexually and they can be supported. Do you understand?

See, what we want to do is to get rid of the whole onion of the polarity itself and just become beings — not male or female; beings — that we share an equal footing with one another. And we can only have in our life what is equal to our God intelligence; not our gender intelligence, our God intelligence. How many of you understand that?

And you women, you are the cleverest of them all.

You know why? Because your energy sits in the third seal. And man's most vulnerable place is his penis, and you know that. You do. The day that you stop going down and gearing down and start gearing up is the day we go home to God. Easy.

And men, the day that they stop living in their penis, in their image, and can at least move to the place of sovereign power — to be able to leave behind their past and know that it is their past — is the day they sit on the same precipice, is the day that they can move into the fourth seal and the fifth seal. But no man ever moves into these kingdoms until he has owned his power and indeed owned that which he thinks he is in terms of his penis and his image. If we were to make every man in this audience a eunuch, who would he be without his manhood? Would he still be able to share the bed with his lover? Would he still be able to share communication? Would he still be able to do that? If he did that, if he were able to do that, then that is a sure sign that he is not his sexuality. And he should never want to be loved but for anything but his true self, of which he himself every day is defining.

New frontiers of self are never-ending. The past of who we are is already known, and it is boring. There is no man in this audience who is more gifted than another man. It is just the way it is. And if they are braggarts, they are fools. I know how men are. Any man who brags about his sexuality is just looking for a harem. You understand? The noble man never does that, and the noble man does not use his sense of sexuality in which to own a woman. Any true man in this audience that is nearer to God will think himself less a man and more God. You understand? The same with you women.

Now what is your morality when it comes to the teaching of what a master is and what a master isn't? So what is a master? A master is one that does not use their body, their face, their breasts, their uterus, their wealth — trying to be skinny, trying to be fat; it doesn't matter — tries not to use that to diminish what they really are. The focus should be what are you as a mind. Mind doesn't really possess gender; did you know that? We don't have in classical science the female mind or the male mind; we only have mind. I say to you it is better to strive to be a mind and have the image of a mind rather than a body, for if you do then, you will join the great and illustrious ranks of masters.

If you always think in terms of competition, if you think in terms of how skinny you are — how many times you miss meals so that you will look the way that you do, how many times you eat so as to pacify what is not given to you — if every time your focus is on your body instead of your mind, you lose. This audience is about being a master. So what is a woman master? One that does not use her body to get what she wants; second, that does not play upon the tragedy of her past to get what she wants; and, third, one who can be who she is from two minutes ago.

Any one of you, and many of you up here, sit and bark and complain about what happened to you in your past. What would you be if you didn't have that memory? Could you stand on your own? Could you? Could you be as beautiful, enthralling, as intriguing, as mindful, if you didn't have to snare a man because of all the terrible things that happened to you? Listen, terrible things happen to everybody. You are not unique. No one here is unique. So would you be able to be as beautiful without a past as you are with one? And if you can eliminate the past and simply be who you are and stand on the merits of your wisdom, then that is something to be proud of. If you can't, you have nothing to be proud of; you are already dead. And any great man who is a master already knows that. You understand?

You cannot entice a master with your victimization. You cannot entice a master with your beauty, with your body. You cannot do that. You only entice a master when you can share equal mind. The morality of women is: Do not use your body to get where you think you are going, and do not use your past to make up where you think your body lacks. Do not control and manipulate someone if you are not in control of yourself — got that? — and to love yourself above all else. And if no one else in this world loves your eyes, loves your face, loves your body, no matter how much you have eaten, no one else loves it but you, that is enough. And anyone after that is more than your fair share. You understand? And then you will be happy. Then you are the rarest amongst jewels.

Most women are never happy until they have got someone in their bed. If you can be happy without any man or woman and simply happy with yourself, you are a jewel beyond price. I would rather be nearer to God than nearer to a man or a woman's heart. So it is said by Christ, "Seek ye first the kingdom of heaven and everything else will be given after you." That is a truth, and to do anything otherwise is to compromise; you are already dead.

Love your children with all your might and with all your heart, and give with them every moment you feel that you were never given to. Languor with them, love with them, and teach them righteously. And never, ever let your children see you insecure, and never, ever show yourself insecure. You take care of that before you ever walk nobly in front of your children. And you teach them how to rectify all problems, and you teach them not prejudice; you teach them love and strength. You teach them that beauty is not everything but nobility and courage are everything. You teach them that who they are must be developed, and that when they are developed to the point of their own acceptance, only then — only then — do they find themselves acceptable to the world and not anytime sooner or later.

You have to teach them that they are good enough and it is they who are here on this journey. You are their mothers. You teach them that. You teach them love and you teach them forgiveness and you teach them righteousness. You do not teach them anything other than that. You do not teach them lies. You do not teach your daughters how to manipulate. You do not teach your daughters to grow up early. You do not teach your sons to grow up early. You teach them to be children, to learn to explore, to learn to love, to learn to understand, to wallow in the innocence of children. And when they come into their adulthood, you teach them responsibility of their bodies but always from the point of view that they are in control — you got that? — and to give them up for the folly of a man is a foolish thing.

It is your hour to be the great teacher. It is your hour to love unconditionally. It is your hour to teach and to love. Never give up your children for any man. Do you hear me? Never. So be it. And I don't care if no one else in the world thinks you are beautiful. I do, and your God does. Don't live for the flesh; live for the mind. And the mind will reward you a millionfold.

Your Highest Compliment — Your Mind, Not Your Body

Now are you listening? So what in the world does this teaching have to do with the Observer and all of those peptides and all of those receptor points that we discussed in the previous Retreat?[5] Everything, because the Observer is impartial. You should know that. The Observer is impartial. And the Observer in how we observe something is impartial to how we will feel it. Are you with me?

Most men and women have always been segregated — and, of course, here we are with a segregated group of women and spattered with a few men — to explain that which is termed the war of the sexes. There isn't any war because basically up until this point everyone has lived by their emotions, their instincts, their bodily feelings. Look, you are in the school of the Great Work. If you were out there on the street tonight he'ing and she'ing, you wouldn't even listen to what I am having to say, though you would wish Monday morning you would have had a few words of wisdom. But tonight, no. You are here to learn.

5 See Candace B. Pert, *Molecules of Emotion* (New York: Simon & Schuster, Inc., 1997).

The Observer in women is no different than the Observer in men. It is just women process the Observer different than men do. The difference is men process it usually and unlayer it all the way to their first seal and women do it to their third seal. That is the difference. And in a world where everything is based on the first three seals, then it is women who have to grapple with that which is termed security. Men grapple with success. Men are not afraid to fail in front of women but they are terrified to fail in front of other men.

So women are the true amazons. They are the real warriors. They know what it is to go out and make war and save family and hearth. They do. That is why their power has been subjugated for eons, because they are a law unto themselves. So what does this have to do with the teaching? And it is simply this: that the Observer in women's greatest caution they have to watch out for is their power over men. And if women would take the power and take it on up instead of down, they would go to their seventh seal easily — easily.

Men with the Observer have a much difficult time because their feelings on anything and everything they create has to do with success, and the success is always anchored in sexuality. Are you listening to me? They have a very hard road. And that hard road is that you can take an enlightened man and put him with a hetaera, and he will drink the waters of forgetfulness nearly all of his life. He will be enslaved by the tiger, and that is when the women always win. I don't care what you say. They always have, except that unfortunately they have never been given the power to lead; they have always done it through their sexuality or through their sons. How many of you understand?

Now in going to become a master, there are men and women masters and they are considered equals; they are not considered unequals. And they have their respective beauty. Men who are masters are beautiful, beautiful, according to the decree of their beauty. Women are breathtaking. They are beautiful according to the decree of their law. But in masters, there is an equalness; there is not an unequalness. There is a sharing. We do not have masters in this realm that live in the first seal and then the others in the fourth seal. They are not masters. They are all on equal bearing. They can only exist in a dominion to where everyone is equal.

So how do women reconcile finally been given equality? Can they still be beautiful and can they still be feminine and still they can be elegant and still be powerful? Yes, there are many who do. Are there women who then, because their beauty has been such a degradation to them, find themselves marred and ugly and that is the way they reach their masterhood? Yes, but don't you know we all understand that. It is called the journey.

And are there men who are virile and beautiful and look like the Gods or the sun God himself? Yes. And are there men who are masters who are ugly and scarred and torn? Yes, because whatever took us there and whatever we cherish is what we get to be, because when we arrive, it has nothing to do with the way we look. It is what we are, the substance of what we are.

Look, I chose a woman's body because they were the most prejudiced group that have ever lived and yet they are the most powerful group; otherwise there would never have been the conspiracy in religion to subvert them. Don't you think I know a sword when I see a sword? And liberating them has been tantamount. Every great prophet that has ever shown its face has been the face of a man, which has left women little to worship and idolize, except maybe nature and herbs and flowers and food and the hearth and their sons. Don't you understand that? Very few women are ever proud of their daughters because in survival they understand the journey. They just do. It is a hard-fought wisdom. I chose a woman because every time I come out here and speak to you, that is the beautiful face you look upon. And can a beautiful face know so much and be so even and be unattached? Can a beautiful face really be God and not be persuaded? Yes. And can it hold power? Absolutely.

Mary, mother of Yeshua ben Joseph, is such a pitiful archetype. No wonder she cries all the time. I want all of you to know that what you can become is like me. You do not have to be a man. You don't have to be a man. All you have to do is be yourself and have your substance, your morals, and your standards be unimpeachable. Then you will be like me.

You can still be as beautiful as you want to be, as ugly as you want to be. You can be as old as you want to be; you can be as young as you want to be. It is all on your terms. The most important thing that you love about me is me, and I cannot be seen. Don't you see? All those times in front of the mirror, and all those foods that you refused to eat, all those things that you overeat, don't you understand this had nothing to do with substance? It is this, and it comes out of the eyes and it is beautiful.

You are that close. Don't use your sexuality to find another husband. Use your God to find yourself. Is that to say then that you are going to be abstinent all through your journey? Maybe. It doesn't really matter if you are already fulfilled. We only need people because we have a lack in ourself. When we are totally fulfilled in ourself, everyone else is company. Do you understand? That is the most desirable woman on the face of the Earth. That is the most desirable woman on the face of the Earth, one who doesn't need anybody. Do you understand me?

You have always anchored downward and you have used your past — the abuses of your past, your culture, your religion, your parents — to hook into someone. And did you know all the time there was a part of you that knew you were doing that? You know that. And you marveled at your cleverness, but you were embarrassed and hated it at the same time because you really felt the things you felt, but yet your head was telling you something else. So who should you listen to, your heart or your head? Your head. And you used that. So you went down and you used your victim to the most, and then when you were ready, you laid the trap of your sexuality. And then to keep them there, you vacillated back to your victim. Are we talking truth here? Oh, yes, we are. And the most beautiful hetaera in here is going to get ugly and old.

So what if you just realized that what you already know here, that is laughing at what you are doing, why don't you follow its advice and go up? What have you got to lose for the next five years? Nothing. What if indeed you just became that which laughs at everything that you do? Why don't you just be that? Don't you know that the Gods from the Seven Sisters[6] will find you because you are not ordinary? And don't you know you will love yourself even more? And don't you know then you can't get rid of these flies because you are so sticky then? Don't you understand that is the way it works? Truth is freedom and it is also seductive. It is the highest compliment we pay ourself. Our body is not our highest compliment; our mind is.

I want you to be great women, all the way to great Gods. I don't want you to be afraid of anything. I don't want you to be afraid of time or your face or wrinkles or fat. I don't want you to be afraid of food. I don't want you to be afraid of poverty. You don't be afraid of any of those because the Observer, that laughs when you are putting this dream together, is the same one that can make you rich, beautiful, and forever young. You got that? So be it.

It is just you have got to be brave enough to strike out on your own. And when you say march and no one else marches with you, you have to go. And if no one is there, stir up your own dust field. Got that? How many of you understand?

Now I daresay if we do a personal reading on all of you, you have been women multitudinous times more beautiful than you are now, uglier than you are now, richer than you are now, poorer than you are now, courtesans, lepers. So what do you have to lose if it doesn't work? Why, you are going to be wiser when you go to the light, and you are just going to create a prettier body because that is all the substance you have gained from it. You

6 The Pleiades.

understand? How many of you understand? So be it.

So now it is no kidding when I told you that the greatest army that ever existed in small part were women. They were the most vicious warriors there ever were. I could hack heads and have no grief. They could do it better than I could because their wrath was unforgivable. That is only to say where they really were and the kind of will that sits underneath their façade, their hypocrisy, their diplomacy.

When you just develop who you are, you will be more beautiful than you ever were before, and you can't be bought, and you can't be flattered, and you can't be sold. You understand? So be it. Then I promise you if you do as I tell you to do, in less than a fortnight you will see the virtue of the teaching. Not only will you no longer be sick in your bodies, because you don't have to keep resorting to your victimization, because it won't be there. So if it is not there, then we don't have those peptides going down to those cells and causing craziness. We don't have disease. And if we have honesty, we don't have to worry about time. So all you have to do is be the core of what you really are, that Observer. And that Observer then will give you immortal life, and you will never die of cancer or any other disease. Women have the greatest cancer associated with their gender because they play these games, and they hate themselves because in the back of their brain someone is laughing the whole time. You got that?

In a fortnight, if you just say the following things:

Let me live what is the voice in my mind.
Let me be it truthfully every moment.
Let me live not on another man's wealth
but on my own mind.
God manifest my mind to wealth, security,
truthfulness,
and enrich my life
that I am a light in the field of the dead.
So be it.

GREAT MEN OF RENOWN

So the men who have come to listen to that which is termed the teachings of an outrageous entity in a woman's body are obviously men of renown. And they are here to listen to truth. They are more than the sum total of that which is termed their first seal. They are vacillating closer to that which is termed the third and onto the fourth. It is just oftentimes you want to define men by their sexuality. You insist upon it, and they acquiesce. But don't you know that their heart is not where their first seal is? If it were, you would have kept them there a long time ago. So the men, as well as the women, are in a move, evolutionarily speaking.

And I want to say on behalf of my beautiful men in this audience that they do have a greater dream, and indeed that they do have a greater desire, and that their ideals for mateship are much loftier than what women give them credit for, for there is not a man in this audience that would not like for that which shares his bed with him and indeed his seed with him that would not be able to share equally, par, a mind that is both challenging, invigorating, and that which is termed a creative Spirit that knows no boundaries and that which, above all, loves God more than they. There is no man in this audience that would not want such a woman and indeed such a mate.

So the men that are here then should not be categorized with that which is termed those who are vulnerable only to hetaerae, because they have come here for another agenda as well, for equally their journey is a journey that is filled with terrors and threats and battles and wars and always the past. And perhaps for a man, the most important of all challenges is failure in the men's eyes around him.

If a man can become greater than the challenges of his counterparts, then he is unequalled. A man who holds his esteem equal to the eyes of the men around him has many equals. So I daresay these beautiful men who are a part of my audience, who come here and indeed who also put down their images and blindfold themselves and sit and blow and cover themselves up and work in the field and toil in the field of God, are not any ordinary men. And if women wanted ordinary men, there is certainly a marketplace to get them.

So then who am I addressing tonight? The point is that it doesn't matter what gender we are. We should never ally ourself to our gender but to our God. And that then speaks of the student on the path of the great Great Work. There is no woman that should beg consideration in the face of masculine attempt. There is no woman here that should say that "I am less because I am a woman and thereby put the responsibility of my care into my male." If you do, you are not in the Great Work. And I daresay, as it were, there is no man here that should say that he is superior to any woman; that he is only equal to mind.

And, remember, the greatest student in this school is a woman, Grandmother. I will put her up against any of you in the field, for some of you are younger and think you are more beautiful and you can get the money of this world. This woman has tied up the kingdom of heaven. She is knocking on the door of heaven, and you are still waiting for someone to approve of how skinny you are. That is the way it is.

I have never considered in this school that men are greater than women. And though I daresay I enjoy the audience of men — I do — I do enjoy the audience of women who have gained a level of mind that I can exchange with. But most women are concerned about their relationships, where they should live, what they should wear, and what they should do, and who they should see. You don't need to consult me to get those answers.

The men of whom I enjoy the company really are

concerned with the path of God; otherwise I wouldn't share their company. I don't find it pleasurable or delightful to talk with empty-headed women. I do not find their face or their bodies appealing if they have no substance. And if they have no mind to articulate righteous questions, I do not find them appealing and neither would anyone else of my stature. What the men of the world would love, the Gods would rebuke. You remember that. And women whose questions are only about their righteous path, creating reality — creating reality staunchly — creating it that their kingdom fulfills them utterly, those are the company of women that I keep because I see them not as women any longer but as Gods, as I do the men that I keep. They are Gods. They are not just men, not just women.

So what does it say about every one of you here. Every one of you here has an Observer. Every one of you are ultimately that. To diminish yourself is to be less than that. To diminish yourself is to become the frailty of your biological, emotional propensities. To be the Observer and to say "I am creating this" and then the next statement is "I am looking forward to the experience" — not that the next statement is "I am creating this but it doesn't feel good to me or it doesn't feel right to me" — I don't want to hear that. A master of the Great Work says, "I am creating. It isn't a matter of how I feel. I will get to that when I manifest it. Anything other than that is just layering the past to my future."

The Retreat is very much about coming down to peeling the onion back, to finding that part that makes us afraid or insecure or unequal or unchallenged or makes us great or ungreat. And if we are going to find the core of who we are, somewhere along the way we must appreciate our beautiful feminine beauty, but it cannot be the end-all to everything. And it is only temporary. Moreover, we cannot get stuck in our penises and our prowess as a lover. And we cannot think that our success is taking another woman away from another man. We cannot think that way. That is the way old satraps think, and they are all dead. Somewhere we must lay that aside and reach for something deeper. We have to go deeper, and we have to find that voice that just observes quietly, unemotionally, and simply is in a state of Isness, that no matter what we put at its feet is not going to make it greater or less.

That is what these Retreats are about, is finding underneath the woman the Observer and being it, being it as boldly as you have been a woman in all your cleverness and in all your manipulation and in all your lies and in all your gearing down for entrapment. And indeed it is finding the Observer in the man who tries and pretends to be brave and strong and spiritual and the breadwinner and sexual. The truth is that really godly men don't enjoy their sexuality that much. They do it for the sake of competition. A truly godly man finds it not on the high end of approval in his physical existence. Anytime you find a man who has more passion for his thought and his creation than he does for his body, you have found a God, and they are rarer than two suns in the sky. That is the journey.

Now why do we say "when you are older and wiser"? Does it mean that physical age must come before wisdom? Usually that is the truth. Why? Because usually that which detracts has finally given way and no one is interested anymore. That is when all of those emotions can finally become wisdom. When nobody cares any longer is when you get really wise. Older-and-wiser is the golden hall of the Gods, but we can become that even when we are in the blush of youth.

This Retreat is about finding the Observer beyond physical sexuality and finding it in a place that it fulfills us utterly — utterly — and that, women, you don't have to play your games anymore. What would you do in a fortnight if you didn't do that? What if instead of making love you told the truth? What if in a fortnight you are really who you were, the Observer; what would happen? Would a lot of things change? Yes, I like it. It is called chaos. They fall away so that something can match to what has presented itself. So who would you be if you couldn't be a hetaera? Do you have the mind? Do you? And about you men: Are you really brave and beautiful without your sexuality? And who are you? Who is with you in your life? That tells you who you are. Could you be that on your own? Could you be honest and truthful? Would you dare to be emotional? Would you dare to tell the truth? Would you dare to do that? In a fortnight if you did, many things would change. And of those of you who nothing would change, then blessed are you, because you already are living the life of righteousness.

And here is the point. We are talking about fabulous wealth that everyone wants. What stands in the way of that? Pretense, hypocrisy, cheating, lying, all of those things that are not the Observer at all. If the Observer can observe fabulous wealth, then how do we create it? Do we put a feminine spin on it or a masculine spin? How are we going to get our wealth? Are we going to get it through a man? Are we going to get it through fight and treachery? How do we get it? Because don't you understand, my beautiful people, that the day the past is over for you is the day that whatever the Observer creates is without the attachment of the past.

What miracle must come into your life but must dress down for your approval? Good point, isn't it, because consciousness and energy is always creating reality, even the emotional body. I want you to be able to create clearly. I want you to create whatever the Observer sees without any ulterior motive. Ulterior motives are the games that men and women play in the fields of God. The clearest, cleanest, fastest way to manifestation is to create without gender. Then it happens straightaway. How many of you understand that? So be it.

If this life were over tomorrow morning, you would go to the light, and you would have a lightbody that looks similar to the one you have but much more beautiful and much more radiant. And if we were to review the lightbody,[7] you wouldn't have a body that was either gender, because who is doing the viewing? That is who we want to be. Got that?

7 The light or life review after death.

So tomorrow you are going to have a woman scientist[8] come and talk to you about emotions; appropriate for a woman to talk to you about. But I want you to remember something in the middle of this dissertation: This is a scientist's point of view. Moreover, it does not explain the great and true self; it only explains the body and its emotions. Got that? And you are going to hear that, as I understand, in my place for two nights. I will see you the next night. Some of you need a scientist to tell you what I have been telling you all along before you accept. Others of you don't need that. It is just knowledge. You add it to your knowledge bank.

There is a circle that even I cannot get into, that I can explain around and around and around. But there is a territory inside of the circle. There are no words in any language nor are there any symbols to be able to explain what is in the circle. It is sort of like the frontal lobe. It is called the quiet area in the brain. It cannot be explained other than it is just quiet. But that is where the seat of consciousness gives its wishes to.

Inside of this circle, I can talk around it and around it and around it — and no one is more gifted in strategy than I am — but there is a place I cannot go into, and that is the place that is necessary for the hierophant to say: I have taught you a discipline. The discipline is to teach you to go to the place that I cannot take you. And the place is — I cannot make you be the Observer nor can I make you hear your own thoughts because you are always busy listening to me. Therein you must enter the circle. The circle is for disciplines and, from the disciplines, self-realization and indeed illumination. You are only going to be illuminated in your true self if you apply what I have taught you, and then you walk into the circle, into

---

8 Candace B. Pert, neuroscientist and research professor in the Department of Physiology and Biophysics at Georgetown University Medical Center in Washington, D.C. She was responsible for the discovery of the opiate receptor in 1972. Her book, *Molecules of Emotion*, presents the findings of her extensive research.

the center nuclei. When you sit in the nuclei, you will see all of your reality. And every discipline I have taught you takes you to that center point. If you do not do that, you will be forever riding the rim of teachings without the experience of truth. And I never came here to deliver teachings without experience. They are hand in hand. The only way you are ever going to grow is to take the teachings and apply them.[9] Got that?

This little Retreat is about entering the circle that is quiet, that no one can explain to you. I have given you the disciplines. It will take you right into the nucleus. If you don't apply them and you don't go there, then you do not deserve the fruit of what the experience will yield to you. None of you do.

Now you want to be a God? I have taught you how to be a God. God is the Observer. How indeed can we be the Observer every moment of every day? You enter the circle and not be afraid to observe the thinking process of the carnal brain that you have created in this lifetime and the reality to which you have created. And at that same nucleus, from the Observer, the Observer has the power to spring forward and grasp any dream in its clutch and make it happen. But that dream can only happen if it is transcendent of one's past, because every day the dream of the image goes on and on and on and on. Got that?

This is the gift of seven years on my rock. This was the gift of my pain. And this was the gift of what happened to me when I left the rock, for I was not the same creature that, wrecked and half-alive, was put there that descended. You are going to enter my rock, and you are going to learn the things that I learned that allowed me to be a changeling and allowed me to be the wind or this woman or that which is termed a sweet caress on your face or the kingdom of heaven. The Observer knows no boundaries. Got that?

---

9 Ramtha's disciplines of the Great Work are practical exercises that allow the student to experience the teachings firsthand. In this case the discipline is called "listening to the voices" and it is simply the act of quieting the body to become acutely aware and observe the continuous stream of thoughts we entertain in our head.

THE GREATEST MYSTERY OF ALL: THE SELF

So, my beloved people, our study in the Ancient School of Wisdom was to study the greatest mystery of all: Who are we? And of course you can never address who we are unless you address that which is termed the intricacies of the biological system to which we call "we" and understand how it works. And of course then, though we can fully analyze it and dissect it and we can see it laugh and cry in life and we see it morbid and cold and stiff in death, we have to ask ourself where lies then the essence that gives it animation and then thereby is gone and has given us only that which is termed the stiff ember, a pitiful remembrance of the animation of life. What is it that gave it animation?

You are not your bodies; if you were, you would go to the grave. And when that undertaker sucks underneath your armpits and between your legs, starts pumping out all the blood of your body down into some sewer on that which is termed a cold, stainless steel gurney, can you really say then, "I was my body"? Because if you were, you are going down the gurney and you are going to the worm, and you are embalmed with chemicals that only preserve an image. But what was it, that delightful entity, that the body was the stage and all of the players that performed the play? Who was it that the body was performing the play for? It is that which has left the throne, and the players have no one to perform for anymore. That is what we call biological death.

So as much as you have heard about the body, simply to educate you that there is no molecule, there is no peptide, there is no hormone in the body that does not carry with it an intent, an information, and that the information is carried to every cell in the body so that the cell can change costumes, and that we have to come back to this point then: Have we really been wrapped up in playing the part too long, have we really taken too seriously our costume, and have we rehearsed the lines too long? So who is the performance for? The entity that you have been practicing to be. And when you listened, who is listening to the voices? That is who you should be, who is listening, not the voices, because that is the eternal. That is the director of the entire escapade.

So what is a master then? A master is one who understands this and understands that the body is coagulated thought, indeed it is coagulated intent. And in its marvelous complexities, its marvelous operation, it is a tribute to who we were, not who we are. Who we are is to challenge who we were, to be who we are. Do you understand? How many of you understand?

The body lives in the past. Who we are is the present. We use the past and challenge the past to become the present. We use a past-coagulated thought from the present in which to exercise our intent. And it is our job to make the past molecule — the past biorhythm, biophysical, bioscience, bioectoplasm — of intent to be our will. And the reason we use it, it brings to the table experience and preparation. And what it lacks we will give to it in the form of will. Where it lacks courage, we will encourage. When we encourage, we change those molecular peptides.

Don't you ever think for one moment that amino acids are stable. They are not. And don't you ever think for one moment that there is some rudimentary law that every day that you wake up that you are pumped full of the same chemicals; you are not. Every one of those molecules are changelings. Every one of them can be changed with attitude and intent. Don't you think for one moment that your DNA is static. It is not. There is a whole lot in junk DNA you have never been and is the potential of becoming that was given to you by the Gods, your progenitors of the neocortex.

Don't you think for one moment that your body is static. It is as pliable as the caterpillar to the butterfly. Any molecule can change with intent because they are only handmaidens of intent. The cells are getting the information. Don't you think for one moment that your cells have a static linear expression. They do not, unless you are dead already consciously; then they are going to follow the biological clock of the DNA in its life expression. And little will the environment ever affect it because the environment is only that which is termed the product of the Observer, and in this case the Observer has simply been emotion. And everyone agrees on that. That is why you have capitalism.

So a master doesn't have a face; only the players in the costume ball have a face. The master — the master — isn't here for pleasure, only the players in the drama reading their script. Only the actors have a script; the viewer doesn't. Are you with me?

So now why do the voices speak to your head? Why do the representatives of the collective body converge in the head and argue for attention? Because they are arguing through the throne of God for precedence, for equitably the continuity of their feelings. And what happens when the God is passive and allows it? Then all you are is the continuity of your emotions. That is all you are.

What happens one day, just like on the Plane of Bliss, when you already know you are doing a light review — you already know that — and you can change anything? What happens the day that you realize that you stop playing the part and become that to which all parts plead for recognition? That is the Lord God of our being. That is what science can never, ever figure out. Science can only study the effect, can only study the phenomenon, can only study the quantum randomness of its expression but can never find the Source. The Source can never explain, be explained by, science; never will be. Never will be.

So when do you become the Observer? In the School of Ancient Wisdom students come to learn to be that, to learn to choose. And they understand that the choice is a great sacrifice because suddenly they are taken out of the spotlight as the drama actors and they are put in the role of the director. Does anyone really want to become what is faceless, what is not out there projected on the screen of quantum potentials? Not any image would want that.

So why are masters so rare? Because it takes a very rarified being to say to themselves, I have got to be more than my senses. There is something more to me than eating, having sex, going to sleep, waking up, romance, integration into society. There has got to be more. And how do I know there is more? Because there is this big hole inside of me that no amount of money or food or sexuality can ever fill. It is a bottomless pit. It is what the Christians call the great Satan. It is a bottomless pit. How can I fill this up? By being it.

There is a part of us that knows that we are noble. So when do you select that? When you stop running these molecules and look at them for being the reason for existence, really and truly, when existence isn't about what you are going to eat, and it isn't about who you are going to seduce, and it isn't about another human being. It is about something that is much more extraordinary than any sensational touch that can be calibrated emotionally in the form of molecular looping to the brain and back to the body, the body back to the brain. You must be more than that.

The School of Ancient Wisdom that always brought about the greatest masters of antiquity are those who were ready to learn to be the Observer without the narcotic effect of emotions — and all emotions are a narcotic — to be that, to make a real clear choice. How many times have I been a man or a woman, and how many times have I had a sexual experience in ten and a half million years? How many bodies have I seen — how many breasts, how many vaginas, how many penises, how many muscles, how much hair, how much face have I seen — in ten and a half million years? How much longer can I duplicate that? When I say I really want to see the cosmos of the Milky Way, do I really mean that? I don't have an emotional hit on the Milky Way but I certainly do on my erection.

The day that you decide to be the Observer, whose dreams can reach the Milky Way, that that is what you want more than the erection, is the day that you will experience the Milky Way. It is the day that you will travel with Gods who really are very grown-up and very mature. The school is about understanding that the molecules of emotion work hand in hand with the progress of the soul and its intent on this plane to make known the unknown and to conquer what is the agitant in the soul, the agitation of an emotion. Look at that. You could be wearing today what you were never able to get over six million years ago. You could be wearing it today in emotions.

How do you get over it? Deciding to be that which doesn't feel anything chemically and to begin to encroach upon the sphere of knowing what it is. And with it comes that which is termed its own momentum of feeling, if you will, that has nothing to do with chemicals: God in its natural state of being — We who fell from Point Zero are the most jolliest of beings. We are the most beautiful of beings. We are without limitation. We are without fear. We are without lack. We are without unhappiness. We are the travelers of time. We have seen it all and done it all. And when we are thoroughly ourself, there is nobody, not even the body of Christ, can possibly magnify our brilliance. There is no molecule, there is no receptor site, indeed there is nothing that can give us what we already are naturally because God is love, and indeed "God is love" is the joy and the glue that holds everything together. The joy is in the glue, not in what is held together. Those are only choices.

And as we then make this journey, we can be assured of one thing: that no matter what comes our way in this life, we are worthy of that opportunity, and that we are equipped — not emotionally crippled but we are equipped — through the will, the scepter of decision, as to what we want. If we simply base every decision upon our emotions, we are doomed and we will never wear the crown of our God, of our Christ. We will never be boldly described as the traveler of time; we will only be another human being, who is never — Heroes: Heroes are the only thing that history ever remembers.

And what is the hero? Simply put, they are the ones that were the rogues against the system. That is why they were remembered. No one remembers all the "yes" people. Do they? No one. No one will ever remember you for being status quo. The only people that are ever remembered are those who listened to another drummer. They were out of step with all humanity. They are what is worth remembering. Shouldn't that be then a sign to you?

So travelers of time are those that have made marks in history. They were never the "yes" man or the "no" woman. They knew it and they did it and let everything fall where it was because they didn't do it for everyone's acceptance. They did it because they were compelled to do it, because they are travelers in time. They did not do it for emotion. If they had done it for emotion, they would never have done it. They would have been intimidated. Do you understand that? And they would never have made the choices they made because it would have cost them their marriage, their relationship. It would have cost them that which is termed their reputation. It would have cost them their gold. It would have cost them their privilege in society. If all of those were on the line and they still made the decision, then they put everything of emotion to the side and made the decision. Those are travelers in time. That is what the Observer is.

Now there are masters that are already in quantum time way beyond you, and you are still here groping about what your mother did to you. You are still fingering yourself with the abandonment of your father. You are still getting sick because no one loved you when you were a child. You are still throwing up at the thought of not being accepted. What kind of children are you going to bear? Neurosis; children who are prone to neurosis, psychosomatic-attitude behavior. That is what kind of children you are bearing. They are going to die early. Nature will take them out in the first plague. They are not equipped for it. They are not emotionally equipped for it. They are not biophysically equipped for it. Do you understand?

To everlasting life
as being the time-traveler,
God I Am,
the Observer
of this blessed life.
So be it.
To life.

THE ULTIMATE SEXUAL EXPERIENCE OF GOD

How many of you are learning? So be it.

Of this, that which is termed this little Retreat, don't you love these little spontaneous events? It takes a lot of baby-sitting to get you to understand nobility. So if you are here, then what does that say about why you came here? That means that there was an aspect of what you learned from some runner that brought you here to further investigate a possibility that could fill up the vacuous self, all of the answers that never existed in society, a runner that would lead you to awakening.

Now you came here because you heard something that rang true somewhere. You don't know where it was. So what emotions happened to you when you heard my name and my word? What happened to you? The face doesn't fit; the body doesn't fit. But something — something — something is problematic in the drama here. The demonstration here is that what you and I are, are equal. The only difference between us is that I know it and you don't know it. And I mean to tell you that it is not simply something that you say tomorrow morning, "I know that I am equal to Ramtha the Enlightened One" — bull — because I have a few tests for you. Let's see if you can do them. No, it is not simply saying the words, because intellectually the brain can do all of those. It can read the parts perfectly. It can. Emotionally doing them is quite another costume indeed. You and I are the same creatures, same divine star, and that we are time-travelers in making known the unknown. We really are. And the divine physics, of course — quantum mechanics, which I adore — is really only a branch to the tree of mathematical understanding of this teaching. It is only a branch, but the trunk of the tree will be found before the year 2000.

Any molecular biologist worth its salt should understand physics and the concept of the Observer and the concept of understanding that that which is termed all particle mass is really coagulated thoughts of energy and that every particle carries an event. And without the marriage of that knowledge, with understanding that which is termed cells and the way that they react and that which is molecules with the way they react, is sort of like playing a part before the third act and not knowing how to finish it. You understand?

Now this is important because it talks about so simply consciousness and energy. And it is the gift that we had when we were created by the Void as Point Zero and then emulated that aspect in creating an aspect of ourself called mirror consciousness. We are the two that is the one that are derived from the eternal. Now we get to choose. We get to choose to either be the DNA fruit of our parents' tree — we get to choose to either be that or that which manipulates it. We get those choices. And it is not as to say that as the Observer, that which is argued before by all emotions, that it simply is without the faculty or the utility to have a sublime feeling. It does. But feelings are overrated. They are overrated, and they are overrated because feelings were originally manufactured for the sake of experiential emotion to an environment that was predestined and preordained by the frontal lobe, as the Observer, willing to be done. Thy will be done.

Feelings give us that which is termed the sensuous copulation of an ideal in that which is termed coagulated mass. We get to copulate. We get to copulate with that which is termed an ideal that has now become mass: It has become a body; it has become an environment, a plane, a challenge. We get to copulate with that. That is the ultimate sexual experience of God. The ultimate sexual experience of God has nothing to do with the propagation of the first seal. It has everything to do with conceiving the fantasy of thought and then copulating it into the environment to bring forth a new child, a new experience, a new law, to which nature then takes them in the engines of ongoing evolution, to take that as a part of the engine, and to evolve and take with you that which is termed that experience, that you are never destroyed in the wake of it.

To a God, copulation is not the sexual spilling of the seed or that which is termed the convulsion of the vagina. The ultimate copulation of a God is to conceive the thought and then to ordain it to be so, as the bride, in reality and then to copulate it through the sensual experience of the body. That is the ultimate sexual experience. It has nothing to do with penises and vaginas. It has everything to do with the loop going back to the brain, to be able to give that satisfying point, that we have experienced ultimately and thoroughly every aspect of the environment, which was originally our idea, and only God has the right to do that. Only a God has the right to do that. It is the ultimate sexual experience.

It is not to say that the Observer is without any faculty or utility of the asset of feeling. But it is not a biological feeling; it is something much grander: a bliss, a euphoric feeling that we get. And the reason that we awaken is because we were drugged by our bodies. We were drugged by that which is termed the illusion of our feelings and never did understand the mechanics behind it when we finally awakened to become that. And here is then the law of the great God. No emotion would be arguing in the brain for preferential treatment to something that is listening, if that which was listening did not hold the ultimate authority of autonomy to be able to make that wish so.

So what is it greater to be: the feeling of pain, of rejection, the feeling of lack? Is it greater to be lack than to be autonomous and the giver of such? Is it greater to feel disease and sickness for the sake of suffering because of the lack of unworthiness? The lack of unworthiness is the incapacity to set upon the throne that which is worthy to sit there to govern the biological systems of our own emotions. We put upon the throne of our intent our sexuality. Our sexuality has not the wisdom to rule our life but its ultimate destruction.

That is why the plagues are killing those who wander

in the fields of such a law, because the virus itself is smarter than those who play in its field. They are not equipped to handle it. You understand? We cannot put upon the throne, we cannot worship the law of suffering more than God. If we worship suffering, then surely goodness and mercy shall not see us through all the days of our life but that we shall bear the open sores of lepers and will be denigrated as that which is old and haggard and become the outcasts of society. And all the money in the world shall not buy us back into what our faded beauty once held for us.

When we worship such emotions, then we worship a fallacy; we do not worship the continuity of life. So what is God? The giver of life. And how do we then define life? An emotional experience. So who gives the emotional experience? God. Who gives nature its boundaries of fruitful womb experience? God. What is nature? Nothing more; the ongoing platform of reality. And who created reality? The God that set the foundations of the world into emotions. That is who sits on the throne that you argue with. That is the Observer. That is the Observer, that I am telling you be the Observer and from the Observer's point of view create the reality. And the reality that you want will fire all sorts of objection from the senate of emotions because they will argue that they feel nothing for this new dream. They feel nothing for it. They will argue.

And should then God listen to emotions? Emotions are only the past. The virgin that sits before the senate — a virgin — has never been penetrated by emotional experience. A virgin thought is the new paradigm, and only when we are becoming the Observer do we have the right then to put forward a new concept and wholly be steadfast in it without feeling anything from it. Do you understand? Because the virgin is that which will give birth to the new heaven and the new Earth. Emotions argue for the old heaven and the old Earth. Turn to your neighbor and explain.

This is the joy and the marvelousness of finding again within ourself our true and most definitive self. This is what we are here — That is what the time-travelers here are all about to do. We can never experience the new kingdom with the old kingdom. It is impossible. The new can never be made from the old unless the old is diminished, washed away, burned in the fire of re-creation. That is the way it is. From the same energy that collapses into a particle, this that collapsed into the old kingdom, the old emotions — and the Observer holds it, holds it, and this argument keeps arguing there in front of the Observer — when it is not given will, it eventually is going to unravel and go back into pure energy with the new program on it, a new consciousness on it, and it will be made anew. Understand? How many of you understand?

So to the human and to human consciousness the temptation is severe. But how much do you want to see through the eyes of a new being, and how much more do you want to see through the window of a new landscape? If what you want to see in your pursuit of a new unknown can withstand that which is termed the destruction of the old, then you are guaranteed to see the new.

What I am teaching you is what all masters will learn, that the journey is the slow mastery of self-deception — self-deception — not only in that which is termed the body but in the environment as well, and in a vicious environment that keeps feeding the emotions. And who has then the ability to destroy the past and all of those? We do. What is our sacrifice? Emotions: whether they are sexual, whether they are suffering, whether they are power, whether they are empathy, they are pity, whether they are hypocrisy, whether they are intellectual denying utterly the physical. These are all stages of mastery and that one by one we must master them. And when we finally do, we will dwell in the house of the Lord forever and ever and ever. And it is from that point then we create the new kingdoms.

To convince the student — to convince the student a lot — is not worthy of the work. We must only teach and convey to who is worthy of the work. Worthiness is already a self-inclination that we are divine but don't have the path in front of us. We know that we are, but we don't know how to get there. You don't have to convince that kind of a student that getting there they will arrive. You don't have to convince them. When you have to convince over and over and over, you have a dead student on your hands. They are dead to their body. They are dead to their past. They are not within the redemption of this lifetime. And it may take a million more lifetimes before they get it. That is why you are so rare.

If you can sacrifice your father's house, your mother's house, if you can sacrifice the womb of your mother which gave you birth — meaning literally if you can sacrifice your genetics — and really overcome your propensities for self-destruction, and create a new module of thought, and that that thought doesn't have any feeling, that is a Christ thought. When it manifests, it will be untainted and the experience will be brand new. Brand new.

Who are such beings? A being that can do this then has the great and remarkable capacity to imagine a kingdom not of this world. They can imagine it without any expectation of feelings because they know they can't feel what is yet to come, and they have learned to do that, and so they can imagine. They can draw new thought-forms and that those new thought-forms are the comforter in their life until that magical moment to where what they have thought manifests, and they get to engage it, to copulate with it. Then they are rewarded. These are the people that have no problem imagining unlimited paradigms, that do not have to be baby-sat with thinking that is positive thinking or thinking that it feels good or that it is wonderful, because you can't say any of that to what is yet to be. It is an unknown. Then these are the masters that have gone on before you. And where have they gone onto? Those places that they imagined and held as the truth. They literally were the beings of God. They were and are the remarkable Observer redeemed in life. So be it.

Now have I told you tonight how much I love you? I do. We have got a march, and it is a long one to catch up with what is ahead of us. I so love you because you are waking up. You are.

Ramtha's Glossary

Analogical. Being analogical means living in the Now. It is the creative moment and is outside of time, the past, and the emotions.

Analogical mind. Analogical mind means one mind. It is the result of the alignment of primary consciousness and secondary consciousness, the Observer and the personality. The fourth, fifth, sixth, and seventh seals of the body are opened in this state of mind. The bands spin in opposite directions, like a wheel within a wheel, creating a powerful vortex that allows the thoughts held in the frontal lobe to coagulate and manifest.

Bands, the. The bands are the two sets of seven frequencies that surround the human body and hold it together. Each of the seven frequency layers of each band corresponds to the seven seals of seven levels of consciousness in the human body. The bands are the auric field that allow the processes of binary and analogical mind.

Binary mind. This term means two minds. It is the mind produced by accessing the knowledge of the human personality and the physical body without accessing our deep subconscious mind. Binary mind relies solely on the knowledge, perception, and thought processes of the neocortex and the first three seals. The fourth, fifth, sixth, and seventh seals remain closed in this state of mind.

Blue Body^{SM}. It is the body that belongs to the fourth plane of existence, the bridge consciousness, and the ultraviolet frequency band. The Blue Body^{SM} is the lord over the lightbody and the physical plane.

Blue Body^{SM} Dance. It is a discipline taught by Ramtha in which the students lift their conscious awareness to the consciousness of the fourth plane. This discipline allows the Blue Body^{SM} to be accessed and the forth seal to be opened.

Blue Body^{SM} Healing. It is a discipline taught by Ramtha in which the students lift their conscious awareness to the consciousness of the fourth plane and the Blue Body^{SM} for the purpose of healing or changing the physical body.

Blue webs. The blue webs represent the basic structure at a subtle level of the physical body. It is the invisible skeletal structure of the physical realm vibrating at the level of ultraviolet frequency.

Body/mind consciousness. Body/mind consciousness is the consciousness that belongs to the physical plane and the human body.

Book of Life. Ramtha refers to the soul as the Book of Life, where the whole journey of involution and evolution of each individual is recorded in the form of wisdom.

C&E^{SM} = R. Consciousness and energy create the nature of reality.

C&E^{SM}. Abbreviation of Consciousness & Energy^{SM}. This is the trademark of the fundamental discipline of manifestation and the raising of consciousness taught in Ramtha's School of Enlightenment. Through this discipline the student learns to create an analogical state of mind, open up its higher seals, and create reality from the Void. A Beginning C&E^{SM} Workshop is the name of the introductory workshop for beginning students in which they learn the fundamental concepts and disciplines of Ramtha's teachings. The teachings of the Beginning C&E^{SM} Workshop can be found in *Ramtha, A Beginner's Guide to Creating Reality,* revised and expanded ed. (Yelm: JZK Publishing, a division of JZK, Inc., 2000), and in *Ramtha: Creating Personal Reality*, Video ed. (Yelm: JZK Publishing, a division of JZK, Inc., 1998).

Christ walk. The Christ walk is a discipline designed by Ramtha in which the student learns to walk very slowly and acutely aware. In this discipline the students learn to manifest, with each step they take, the mind of a Christ.

Consciousness. Consciousness is the child who was born from the Void's contemplation of itself. It is the essence and fabric of all being. Everything that exists originated in consciousness and manifested outwardly through its handmaiden energy. A stream of consciousness refers to the continuum of the mind of God.

Consciousness and energy. Consciousness and energy are the dynamic force of creation and are inextricably combined. Everything that exists originated in consciousness and manifested through the modulation of its energy impact into mass.

Disciplines of the Great Work. Ramtha's School of Ancient Wisdom is dedicated to the Great Work. The disciplines of the Great Work practiced in Ramtha's School of Enlightenment are all designed in their entirety by Ramtha. These practices are powerful initiations where the student has the opportunity to apply and experience firsthand the teachings of Ramtha.

Emotions. An emotion is the physical, biochemical effect of an experience. Emotions belong to the past, for they are the expression of experiences that are already known and mapped in the neuropathways of the brain.

Energy. Energy is the counterpart of consciousness. All consciousness carries with it a dynamic energy impact, radiation, or natural expression of itself. Likewise, all forms of energy carry with it a consciousness that defines it.

Enlightenment. Enlightenment is the full realization of the human person, the attainment of immortality, and unlimited mind. It is the result of raising the kundalini energy sitting at the base of the spine to the seventh seal that opens the dormant parts of the brain. When the energy penetrates the lower cerebellum and the midbrain, and the subconscious mind is opened, the individual experiences a blinding flash of light called enlightenment.

Evolution. Evolution is the journey back home from the slowest levels of frequency and mass to the highest levels of consciousness and Point Zero.

Fieldwork^{SM}. Fieldwork^{SM} is one of the fundamental disciplines of Ramtha's School of Enlightenment. The students are taught to create a symbol of something they want to know and experience and draw it on a paper card. These cards are placed with the blank side facing out on the fence rails of a large field. The students blindfold themselves and focus on their symbol, allowing their body to walk freely to find their card through the application of the law of consciousness and energy and analogical mind.

Fifth plane. The fifth plane of existence is the plane of superconsciousness and x-ray frequency. It is also known as the Golden Plane or paradise.

Fifth seal. The fifth seal is the center of our spiritual body that connects us to the fifth plane. This seal is associated with the thyroid gland and with speaking and living the truth without dualism.

First plane. It refers to the material or physical plane. It is the plane of the image consciousness and Hertzian frequency. It is the lowest and densest form of coagulated consciousness and energy.

First seal. The first seal is associated with the reproductive organs, sexuality, and survival.

First three seals. The first three seals are the seals of sexuality, survival, pain and suffering, victimization, and tyranny. These are the seals commonly at play in all of the complexities of the human drama.

Fourth plane. The fourth plane of existence is the realm of the bridge consciousness and ultraviolet frequency. This plane is described as the plane of Shiva, the destroyer of the old and creator of the new. In this plane, energy is not yet split into positive and negative charge. Any lasting changes or healing of the physical body must be changed first at the level of the fourth plane and the Blue Body^{SM}. This plane is also called the Blue Plane, or the plane of Shiva.

Fourth seal. The fourth seal is associated with unconditional love and the thymus gland. When this seal is activated, a hormone is released that maintains the body in perfect health and stops the aging process.

God. Ramtha's teachings are an exposition of the statement, "You are God." Humanity is described as the forgotten Gods. God is different from the Void. God is the point of awareness that sprang from the Void contemplating itself. It is consciousness and energy exploring and making known the unknown potentials of the Void. It is the omnipotent and omnipresent essence of all creation.

God within. It is the Observer, the true self, the primary consciousness, the Spirit, the God within the human person.

God/man. The full realization of a human being.

God/woman. The full realization of a human being.

Gods. The Gods are technologically advanced beings from other star systems who came to Earth 455,000 years ago. These Gods manipulated the human race genetically, mixing and modifying our DNA with theirs. They are responsible for the evolution of the neocortex and used the human race as a subdued work force. Evidence of these events is recorded in the Sumerian tablets and artifacts. This term is also used to describe the true identity of humanity, the forgotten Gods.

Golden body. It is the body that belongs to the fifth plane, superconsciousness, and x-ray frequency.

Great Work. The Great Work is the practical application of the teachings of the Schools of Ancient Wisdom. It refers to the disciplines by which the human person becomes enlightened and is transmuted into an immortal, divine being.

Hierophant. A hierophant is a master teacher who is able to manifest what they teach and initiate their students into such knowledge.

Hyperconsciousness. Hyperconsciousness is the consciousness of the sixth plane and gamma ray frequency.

Infinite Unknown. It is the frequency band of the seventh plane of existence and ultraconsciousness.

Involution. Involution is the journey from Point Zero and the seventh plane to the slowest and densest levels of frequency and mass.

JZ Knight. JZ Knight is the only person appointed by Ramtha to channel him. Ramtha refers to JZ as his beloved daughter. She was Ramaya, the eldest of the children given to Ramtha during his lifetime.

Kundalini. Kundalini energy is the life force of a person that descends from the higher seals to the base of the spine at puberty. It is a large packet of energy reserved for human evolution, commonly pictured as a coiled serpent that sits at the base of the spine. This energy is different from the energy coming out of the first three seals responsible for sexuality, pain and suffering, power, and victimization. It is commonly described as the sleeping serpent or the sleeping dragon. The journey of the kundalini energy to the crown of the head is called the journey of enlightenment. This journey takes place when this serpent wakes up and starts to split and dance around the spine, ionizing the spinal fluid and changing its molecular structure. This action causes the opening of the midbrain and the door to the subconscious mind.

Life force. The life force is the Father, the Spirit, the breath of life within the person that is the platform from which the person creates its illusions, imagination, and dreams.

Life review. It is the review of the previous incarnation that occurs when the person reaches the third plane after death. The person gets the opportunity to be the Observer, the actor, and the recipient of its own actions. The unresolved issues from that lifetime that emerge at the life review set the agenda for the next incarnation.

Light, the. The light refers to the third plane of existence.

Lightbody. It is the same as the radiant body. It is the body that belongs to the third plane of conscious awareness and the visible light frequency band.

List, the. The List is the discipline taught by Ramtha where the student gets to write a list of items they desire to know and experience and then learn to focus on it in an analogical state of consciousness. The List is the map used to design, change, and reprogram the neuronet of the person. It is the tool that helps to bring meaningful and lasting changes in the person and their reality.

Make known the unknown. This phrase expresses the original divine mandate given to the Source consciousness to manifest and bring to conscious awareness all of the infinite potentials of the Void. This statement represents the basic intent that inspires the dynamic process of evolution.

Mind. Mind is the product of streams of consciousness and energy acting on the brain creating thought forms, holographic segments, or neurosynaptic patterns called memory. The streams of consciousness and energy are what keep the brain alive. They are its power source. A person's ability to think is what gives them a mind.

Mind of God. The mind of God comprises the mind and wisdom of every lifeform that ever lived on any dimension, in any time, or that ever will live on any planet or any star.

Monkey-mind. Monkey-mind refers to the flickering mind of the personality.

Mother/Father Principle. It is the source of all life, God the Father, the eternal Mother, the Void.

Name-field. The name-field is the name of the large field where the discipline of Fieldwork^{SM} is practiced.

Observer. It refers to the Observer responsible for collapsing the particle/wave of quantum mechanics. It represents the true self, the Spirit, primary consciousness, the God within the human person.

Outrageous. Ramtha uses this word in a positive way to express something or someone who is extraordinary and unusual, unrestrained in action, and excessively bold or fierce.

People, places, things, times, and events. These are the main areas of human experience to which the personality is emotionally attached. These areas represent the past of the human person and constitute the content of the emotional body.

Plane of Bliss. It refers to the plane of rest where souls get to plan their next incarnations after their life reviews. It is also known as heaven and paradise where there is no suffering, no pain, no need or lack, and where every wish is immediately manifested.

Plane of demonstration. The physical plane is also called the plane of demonstration. It is the plane where the person has the opportunity to demonstrate its creative potentiality in mass and witness consciousness in material form in order to expand its emotional understanding.

Point Zero. It refers to the original point of awareness created by the Void through its act of contemplating itself. Point Zero is the original child of the Void.

Ram. Ram is a shorter version of the name Ramtha. Ramtha means the Father.

Ramaya. Ramtha refers to JZ Knight as his beloved daughter. She was Ramaya, the first one to become Ramtha's adopted child during his lifetime. Ramtha found Ramaya abandoned on the steppes of Russia. Many people gave their children to Ramtha during the march as a gesture of love and highest respect; these children were to be raised in the House of the Ram. His children grew to the great number of 133 even though he never had offspring of his own blood.

Ramtha (etymology). The name of Ramtha the Enlightened One, Lord of the Wind, means the Father. It also refers to the Ram who descended from the mountain on what is known as the Terrible Day of the Ram. "It is about that in all antiquity. And in ancient Egypt, there is an avenue dedicated to the Ram, the great conqueror. And they were wise enough to understand that whoever could walk down the avenue of the Ram could conquer the wind." The word Aram, the name of Noah's grandson, is formed from the Aramaic noun Araa — meaning earth, landmass — and the word Ramtha, meaning high. This Semitic name echoes Ramtha's descent from the high mountain, which began the great march.

Runner. A runner in Ramtha's lifetime was responsible for bringing specific messages or information. A master teacher has the ability to send runners to other people that manifest their words or intent in the form of an experience or an event.

Second plane. It is the plane of existence of social consciousness and the infrared frequency band. It is associated with pain and suffering. This plane is the negative polarity of the third plane of visible light frequency.

Second seal. This seal is the energy center of social consciousness and the infrared frequency band. It is associated with pain and suffering and is located in the lower abdominal area.

Self, the. The self is the true identity of the human person. It is the transcendental aspect of the person. It refers to the Observer, the primary consciousness.

Sending-and-receiving. Sending-and-receiving is the name of the discipline taught by Ramtha in which the student learns to access information using the faculties of the midbrain to the exclusion of sensory perception. This discipline develops the student's psychic ability of telepathy and divination.

Seven seals. The seven seals are powerful energy centers that constitute seven levels of consciousness in the human body. The bands are the way in which the physical body is held together according to these seals. In every human being there is energy spiraling out of the first three seals or centers. The energy pulsating out of the first three seals manifests itself respectively as sexuality, pain, or power. When the upper seals are unlocked, a higher level of awareness is activated.

Seventh plane. The seventh plane is the plane of ultraconsciousness and the Infinite Unknown frequency band. This plane is where the journey of involution began. This plane was created by Point Zero when it imitated the act of contemplation of the Void and the mirror or secondary consciousness was created. A plane of existence or dimension of space and time exists between two points of consciousness. All the other planes were created by slowing down the time and frequency band of the seventh plane.

Seventh seal. This seal is associated with the crown of the head, the pituitary gland, and the attainment of enlightenment.

Shiva. The Lord God Shiva represents the Lord of the Blue Plane and the Blue Body^SM. Shiva is not used in reference to a singular deity from Hinduism. It is rather the representation of a state of consciousness that belongs to the fourth plane, the ultraviolet frequency band, and the opening of the fourth seal. Shiva is neither male nor female. It is an androgynous being, for the energy of the fourth plane has not yet been split into positive and negative polarity. This is an important distinction from the traditional Hindu representation of Shiva as a male deity who has a wife. The tiger skin at its feet, the trident staff, and the sun and the moon at the level of the head represent the mastery of this body over the first three seals of consciousness. The kundalini energy is pictured as fiery energy shooting from the base of the spine through the head. This is another distinction from some Hindu representations of Shiva with the serpent energy coming out at the level of the fifth seal or throat. Another symbolic image of Shiva is the long threads of dark hair and an abundance of pearl necklaces, which represent its richness of experience owned into wisdom. The quiver and bow and arrows are the agent by which Shiva shoots its powerful will and destroys imperfection and creates the new.

Sixth plane. The sixth plane is the realm of hyperconsciousness and the gamma ray frequency band. In this plane the awareness of being one with the whole of life is experienced.

Sixth seal. This seal is associated with the pineal gland and the gamma ray frequency band. The reticular formation that filters and veils the knowingness of the subconscious mind is opened when this seal is activated. The opening of the brain refers to the opening of this seal and the activation of its consciousness and energy.

Social consciousness. It is the consciousness of the second plane and the infrared frequency band. It is also called the image of the human personality and the mind of the first three seals. Social consciousness refers to the collective consciousness of human society. It is the collection of thoughts, assumptions, judgments, prejudices, laws, morality, values, attitudes, ideals, and emotions of the fraternity of the human race.

Soul. Ramtha refers to the soul as the Book of Life, where the whole journey of involution and evolution of the individual is recorded in the form of wisdom.

Subconscious mind. The seat of the subconscious mind is the lower cerebellum or reptilian brain. This part of the brain has its own independent connections to the frontal lobe and the whole of the body and has the power to access the mind of God, the wisdom of the ages.

Superconsciousness. This is the consciousness of the fifth plane and the x-ray frequency band.

Tahumo. Tahumo is the discipline taught by Ramtha in which the student learns the ability to master the effects of the natural environment — cold and heat — on the human body.

Tank field. It is the name of the large field with the labyrinth that is used for the discipline of The Tank^{SM}.

Tank^{SM}, The. It is the name given to the labyrinth used as part of the disciplines of Ramtha's School of Enlightenment. The students are taught to find the entry to this labyrinth blindfolded and move through it focusing on the Void without touching the walls or using the eyes or the senses. The objective of this discipline is to find, blindfolded, the center of the labyrinth or a room designated and representative of the Void.

Third plane. This is the plane of conscious awareness and the visible light frequency band. It is also known as the light plane and the mental plane. When the energy of the Blue Plane is lowered down to this frequency band, it splits into positive and negative polarity. It is at this point that the soul splits into two, giving origin to the phenomenon of soulmates.

Third seal. This seal is the energy center of conscious awareness and the visible light frequency band. It is associated with control, tyranny, victimization, and power. It is located in the region of the solar plexus.

Thought. Thought is different from consciousness. The brain processes a stream of consciousness modifying it into segments — holographic pictures — of neurological, electrical, and chemical prints called thoughts. Thoughts are the building blocks of mind.

Twilight™ ^{SM}. This term is used to describe the discipline taught by Ramtha in which the students learn to put their bodies in a catatonic state similar to deep sleep, yet retaining their conscious awareness.

Twilight™ ^{SM} Visualization Process. It is the process used to practice the discipline of the List or other visualization formats.

Ultraconsciousness. It is the consciousness of the seventh plane and the Infinite Unknown frequency band. It is the consciousness of an ascended master.

Unknown God. The Unknown God was the single God of Ramtha's ancestors, the Lemurians. The Unknown God also represents the forgotten divinity and divine origin of the human person.

Upper four seals. The upper four seals are the fourth, fifth, sixth, and seventh seals.

Void, the. The Void is defined as one vast nothing materially, yet all things potentially.

Yellow brain. The yellow brain is Ramtha's name for the neocortex, the house of analytical and emotional thought. The reason why it is called the yellow brain is because the neocortices were colored yellow in the original two-dimensional, caricature-style drawing Ramtha used for his teaching on the function of the brain and its processes. He explained that the different aspects of the brain in this particular drawing are exaggerated and colorfully highlighted for the sake of study and understanding. This specific drawing became the standard tool used in all the subsequent teachings on the brain.

Yeshua ben Joseph. Ramtha refers to Jesus Christ by the name Yeshua ben Joseph, following the Jewish traditions of that time.

FIG. A: THE SEVEN SEALS:
SEVEN LEVELS OF CONSCIOUSNESS IN THE HUMAN BODY

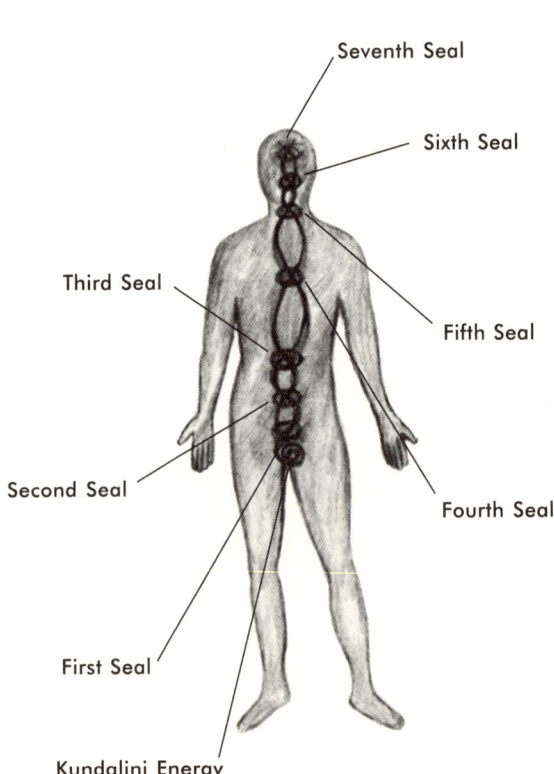

Seventh Seal

Sixth Seal

Third Seal

Fifth Seal

Second Seal

Fourth Seal

First Seal

Kundalini Energy

Fig. B: Seven Levels of Consciousness and Energy

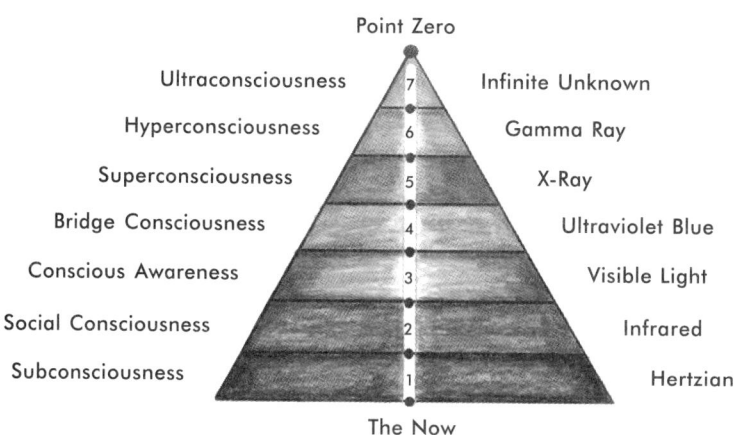

Fig. C: The Brain

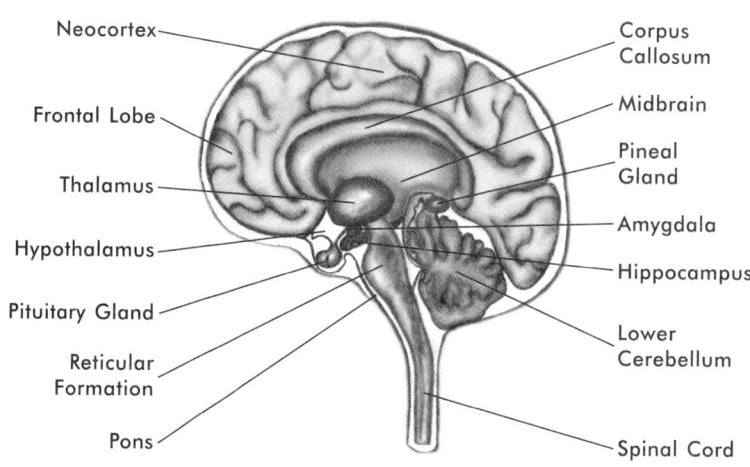

Ramtha's School of Enlightenment,
THE SCHOOL OF ANCIENT WISDOM

A Division of JZK, Inc.
P.O. Box 1210
Yelm, Washington 98597
360.458.5201
800.347.0439
www.ramtha.com
www.jzkpublishing.com